DO NOT REMOVE
CARDS FROM POCKET

CHILDBEARING

A Book of Choices

Other books by Gene R. Hawes

THE CAREER-CHANGER'S SOURCEBOOK

THE COLLEGE BOARD GUIDE TO GOING
TO COLLEGE WHILE WORKING

SPEAK FOR SUCCESS
(with Eugene Ehrlich)

HAWES ON GETTING INTO COLLEGE

HAWES GUIDE TO SUCCESSFUL STUDY SKILLS
(with Lynne Salop Hawes)

HOW TO RAISE YOUR CHILD TO BE A WINNER
(with Helen G. and Martin S. Weiss)

HAWES COMPREHENSIVE GUIDE TO COLLEGES

EDUCATIONAL TESTING FOR THE MILLIONS

THE OUTDOOR CAREERS GUIDE
(with Douglass M. Brownstone)

THE ENCYCLOPEDIA OF SECOND CAREERS

THE COLLEGE MONEY BOOK
(with David M. Brownstone)

GETTING COLLEGE COURSE CREDITS BY EXAMINATION
TO SAVE DOLLARS

THE CONCISE DICTIONARY OF EDUCATION
(with Lynne Salop Hawes)

THE COMPLETE CAREER GUIDE
(with David M. Brownstone)

CAREERS TOMORROW: LEADING GROWTH FIELDS FOR
COLLEGE GRADUATES

CAREERS TODAY: LEADING GROWTH FIELDS ENTERED BY
SHORT TRAINING
(with Mark Hawes and Christine Fleming)

COLLEGE ON YOUR OWN
(with Gail Thain Parker)

THE NEW AMERICAN GUIDE TO COLLEGES

COLLEGE LEARNING ANYTIME, ANYWHERE
(with Ewald Nyquist and Jack Arbolino)

HOW TO GET COLLEGE SCHOLARSHIPS

STUDENT'S GUIDE TO STUDY IN THE U.S.A.

CHILDBEARING

A Book of Choices

by

Ruth Watson Lubic, C.N.M., Ed.D.
General Director, Maternity Center Association

Gene R. Hawes

A Hudson Group Book

McGraw-Hill Book Company
New York St. Louis San Francisco Toronto Hamburg Mexico

To my husband, Bill,
who fathered not only Douglas
but my career and this book.

R. W. L.

Figures in Chapter 5 (Figures 5.1, 5.3) and in Chapters 7 (Figures 7.4–7.11) and 10 are reprinted by permission of Maternity Center Association from *Preparation for Childbearing, Fifth Edition,* 1985, copyright © by Maternity Center Association.

1 2 3 4 5 6 7 8 9   DOCDOC   8 7 6

ISBN 0-07-038908-X

LIBRARY OF CONGRESS CATALOGING-IN-PUBLICATION DATA

Lubic, Ruth Watson.
  Childbearing: a book of alternatives.
  Bibliography: p.
  Includes index.
  1. Pregnancy.   2. Childbirth.   I. Hawes, Gene R.
II. Title. [DNLM: 1. Delivery—popular works.
2. Pregnancy—popular works. WQ 150 L929c]
RG525.L83 1986   618.2   86-7341
ISBN 0-07-038908-X

Book design by M. R. P. Design

Acknowledgments

The acknowledgments for any book usually include those near and dear, spouses, children and parents who suffer with the authors the labor of production, much as do the support persons you will read about in these pages and be encouraged to employ. Our thanks extend beyond these persons both back and forward in time. Historically, the Board of Directors of Maternity Center Association deserve much of the credit for making the central theme of this book about childbearing—choices—available to families. Particular thanks go to Mrs. Walter M. Rothschild, Mary P. Oenslager, Phyllis Farley, Katherine S. J. Law and Jane L. Powell. Other thanks must be given those people who breathed life into the concept of nurse-midwifery and family centered birth and demonstrated the professional behaviors which Dr. Lubic has endeavored to emulate: Hazel Corbin, Marion Strachan, Ruth Beeman and Edith Wonnell. The creative and indefatigable Kitty Ernst is a very special model, colleague and friend. Rosemary Diulio has been exceptionally important to this book. The wonderful staff of the Childbearing Center, nurse-midwives, physicians, nurse-midwife assistants and all their indispensable support personnel, has shown good cheer, stamina and unfailing clinical excellence in making the birth center concept a reality. Our physician advisors deserve special recognition for their visionary support.

The most deserving of appreciation, however, are those courageous families of past, present and future who did and do believe enough in the inherent normalcy of pregnancy and birth to participate in health care innovation, in spite of controversy. To them should go the greatest share of credit, for without them, the served, there is no service.

Individuals and couples who were extremely helpful to Mr. Hawes in particular in his co-authorship of the book included Frances Luppi, who assisted with the research and early drafting of Chapter 15, "The Baby's First Few Weeks," and David Merrill, who similarly assisted with Chapter 4, "Weight Gain and Nutrition."

Among other persons who helped Mr. Hawes by providing invaluable understanding of their own childbearing experiences were: Monica and Mark Hawes, Roberta and Robert Teller, Elizabeth and Charles Settens, Gayle and Christopher Rice, and Andrea and Robert Terdiman. Such persons included as well these classmates of Mr. Hawes at a Maternity Center Association class for expectant first-time parents: Christine and Charles Bardach, Maria and Otto Caveda, Belle and Michael Cheverino, Robin Blair Fetter and Frank Fetter, Susan Freston-Hermann and Eric Hermann, Germaine and Joseph Johnson, Yvonne and Mithra Neuman, and Joanne and Richard Schmitt. Mr. Hawes is also very grateful to the instructor of that class, Rosemary Diulio.

Contents

・ *Contents* ・

III. *Birth and Early Parenting* / *195*

IV. *Birth with Special Problems* / *265*

Appendices / *303*

Introduction: Is There One Best Way of Having a Baby?

Of course the answer to this question is "no." There is no one childbirth method which is best for all women. Women differ in their physical, psychological, cultural, and spiritual makeup and needs.

Most women will be able to experience a normal vaginal birth. Some will have a clear need for surgical intervention. For that majority who can experience birth as a normal health event, a variety of options are available. In general, these choices reflect the two approaches taken by maternity care providers.

In one approach, the provider makes most of the decisions, with limited input and responsibility on the part of the woman and her family. This usually involves greater use of technology in the form of diagnostic tools during pregnancy, and of chemical and/or surgical techniques during labor and delivery. At the core of this approach is the belief that pregnancy and birth are less physiologic than pathologic and therefore must be actively controlled and managed by experts.

The other approach treats pregnancy and birth as normal physiologic events, the successful monitoring of which requires an active decision-making role on the part of the expectant woman and her family. This approach does not reject the use of technology, but applies it only when there is a demonstrated need. The responsibility of the childbearing woman as a partner in a team is emphasized.

Your first decision, then, concerns the role you want to have: whether you elect to be relatively passive or relatively active in the management of your pregnancy and childbirth. In this book the latter approach will be emphasized because, quite frankly, it is our belief that, in order to be effective, health care must freely involve the persons who need or seek the assistance of professionals. The equation for reproductive health can be complete only when experts in knowing their own bodies—women—interact with experts in the conditions of pregnancy and birth (physicians, nurse-midwives, nurses, nutritionists, parent educators, social workers, and others).

Recent advances in childbearing offer you many options. Consumer advocate Diony Young states in *Changing Childbirth* that the decade of the 1970s "witnessed an extraordinary humanistic and technological revolution in obstetrical and newborn care." [1] As a result of that revolution, alternatives have become available which were undreamed-of twenty-five years ago, with the result that childbearing today is more emotionally rewarding for the whole family—as well as far more healthy for mother and baby. These developments include the introduction of natural childbirth; the Dick-Read, Lamaze, and Bradley methods for participation in labor and birth; family-centered childbirth; the Leboyer approach of "gentle birth" for the baby; the principles of infant bonding; and alternative birth settings. The growing availability of nurse-midwives, who serve as team members with obstetricians and who place a great value on the expression of feelings as well as high-quality physical care for healthy women, is another recent change.

You will also have choices to make among many powerful new methods of diagnosis and treatment, the results of technologic breakthroughs of recent years. These can give you and your unborn baby greater protection than ever before from rare but very serious hazards. Examples include amniocentesis, ultrasonography, electronic fetal monitoring, and neonatal intensive-care units.

In general, these two approaches—the humanistic and the technologic—have attracted strong advocates on either side, with a resulting polarization between the conventional doctor/hospital system and some families, and among health-care professionals as well.

Whichever approach you choose, finding a professional with a philosophy similar to your own is crucial. It follows that you must assess your feelings, get the information you need to fill any gaps in your knowledge, and then come to a conclusion about the best way of birth for you.

Attaining a balanced understanding of the wide range of options in childbearing can be difficult, because a number of the recent epochal advances have generated sharp controversy among medical authorities and health professionals. Our aim is to help you learn about all the opportunities open to you and to help you gain the knowledge you need to choose freely and wisely in making your decisions.

A deep conviction of ours gives rise to this aim: When you're well informed, the one best way of having your baby is the one on which you decide.

I

Pregnancy

1

Where Your Decisions Begin

In assessing your own philosophy about childbearing, you will naturally think back to your earliest impressions of pregnancy and birth. These impressions come from many sources—the media, sex education programs in school or religious institutions, and discussions with friends and family members.

In all likelihood, your own mother's experiences and attitudes will influence you most strongly, either positively or negatively. Even if she never talked about pregnancy and birth directly, feeling-tones and body language communicate themselves readily, especially to girls. Girls recognize early on that their mothers are "girls" too.

What happened, for example, when you passed a pregnant woman on the street and for the first time asked about her shape? Was the question avoided, answered with a tone of embarrassment or envy, or answered with a positive feeling?

Did you overhear your mother and father or other family members discussing unwanted pregnancies? Did accusations about pain suffered in labor surface in arguments? Did your father express his feelings about pregnancy and birth?

Does your mother react with joy to questions about your own birth? Or does she seem to have had a difficult time, or possibly express resentment or regret at the way you and she were treated in the hospital setting? Stories of breastfeeding failure, for example, are common among women who had babies in the 1940s, '50s, and '60s, when mothers and babies were together in the hospital only for brief scheduled feedings.

3

Do you have younger siblings? Do you remember your mother's behavior during her pregnancies? Did these new arrivals in your family cause jealousy and resentment on your part? Have your siblings borne children or become fathers themselves?

The answers to these questions will help you clarify your current feelings about childbearing.

Decisions You Can Make Today

After clarifying your current attitude, you can begin to fill in any information gaps. There are several important decisions you can make about your own childbearing experience:

Do you want to be conscious and participating, physically and emotionally, during childbirth? You can choose to go through the familiar, conventional childbirth experience in which you will be "delivered," often under anesthesia. Or instead, you can choose to "give birth" with little or no anesthetics or analgesics (if you're likely to have a normal birth, as most pregnant women are).

If you make the choice to have little or no medication, you and your partner can attend classes in which you will learn exercises to develop your physical fitness for doing your part in giving birth, self-help techniques for making yourself comfortable during pregnancy and for relieving pain during labor, and methods of support which enable your partner to provide physical and emotional comfort during labor and birth.

If you should decide to have your baby with little or no anesthesia or analgesics, you're likely to do so for three main reasons:

- You'd like to avoid chemicals that can be hazardous to your unborn baby.
- You want to have the complete, authentic experience of giving birth to your child, as a natural and healthy event.
- You have learned from others that having a baby in this way is both possible and rewarding—and that, on the other hand, analgesics and anesthetics can cause "hangovers" with uncomfortable after-effects.

Would you like to have the baby's father or another person present and actively helping during labor and birth? Today you can decide to have your baby's father share in the actual labor and childbirth, instead of having him separated from you until you're back in your

4

hospital room. Or you might choose another family member or a close friend as the partner to be with you for the birth. In many hospitals today, partners who take part in prenatal classes can stay all through labor and delivery—and in some cases even through a surgical delivery by cesarean section.

Do you want a homelike setting for labor and birth? You can choose between traditional labor and delivery rooms in a hospital (the latter much like an operating room) and rooms resembling bedrooms, outfitted for the comfort of family members. In a few hospitals, you may find alternative birth centers which also provide sitting-room and kitchen facilities. Homelike environments such as this are provided increasingly in hospitals, as well as in the out-of-hospital birth centers which they copy.

Do you want your newborn baby to be given to you for holding and "bonding" right after birth? You can choose traditional birth arrangements, in which the baby is cared for separately by nursing personnel at birth. Or you can choose approaches in which you and your partner hold, cuddle, bathe, and generally welcome your infant to the outer world. Experts feel that such "bonding" at birth can have profound, permanent, and positive consequences for both the infant and the parents.

Do you want the baby to be allowed to stay with you? You may choose to have your baby at a hospital where the infant is kept in the hospital nursery most of the time, or at a hospital or birth center where the baby stays with the mother in a rooming-in unit. Full or partial rooming-in is possible at many hospitals.

Do you want to leave the birth setting only a few hours after the birth? Out-of-hospital birth centers feature early discharges (twelve to twenty-four hours after birth) and spend time in the prenatal period preparing parents to take their baby home early. Increasingly, hospitals also are providing this option, particularly as cost-consciousness rises.

Do you want to select an alternative health-care specialist or child-birth facility for prenatal care and the birth? For your childbearing care-giver, you can choose among the following types of professionals, who are formally educated to provide such care:

- M.D.'s (Doctors of Medicine) or D.O.'s (Doctors of Osteopathy) who are board-certified in obstetrics and gynecology; they have had long specialty training in the management of complicated childbearing and in surgical procedures like the cesarean section.
- M.D.'s or D.O.'s who limit their practice to obstetrics and gynecology and who usually have surgical privileges at hospitals.

- M.D.'s and D.O.'s who are general or family practitioners, and who sometimes do not have surgical privileges at hospitals.
- C.N.M.'s (Certified Nurse-Midwives) who are specialists in normal, healthy childbearing and who have access to obstetrical consultation.

Still more care-giver choices may be open to you. Some states license other professionals, such as chiropractors and naturopaths, to provide maternity care and attend births. In addition, a number of states also license persons who may or may not have had professional education and training in maternity care and birth; these care-givers are usually called lay midwives, empiric midwives, or traditional birth attendants.

Facilities from which you can choose include hospitals (with differing childbirth practices), out-of-hospital birth centers, and your home.

Your choice of type of care-provider and facility is a basic decision which may determine your answers to the questions we list.

Is It Better to Let Your Care-giver Make the Decisions?

Most of us have been conditioned to think that the experts know best. That may be true in illness (although options in treatment are being presented more and more, even to persons who are critically ill and to their families). But making your own decisions about healthy childbearing may prove genuinely satisfying for you. Many expectant parents today find such decision-making exciting and confidence-building. In their eyes, childbearing is not an illness for a professional specialist to control, but rather a natural body function that they can actively guide and experience. You and your partner could find it rewarding to be completely aware of and involved in the process of bringing your baby into the world. However, your decision to try such an approach should be based on sufficient information, consultation and discussion.

The extent to which you should get involved in making your own childbearing decisions is a controversial issue. Some parents and experts urge very active involvement. We are among them. In this approach, you learn enough to take shared responsibility with the care-giver in carrying out your prenatal care and your childbirth experience. Typically, you may also plan on birth at a birth center or even at home (if your physical condition and health history indicate you're likely to have a normal, low-risk birth).

Experts at the opposite end of the spectrum recommend conventional childbearing care. In their approach, you learn a number of facts about pregnancy and labor and decide on a conventional hospital birth. You then turn over the greater part of all subsequent decisions concerning prenatal care and birth to your care-giver—who would typically be an M.D. specializing in obstetrics.

Are There Advantages to Making Your Own Decisions?

In our experience, learning how to make decisions during pregnancy and birth will realize other special advantages. For example, it can help you develop a whole new sense of self-confidence in taking care of your own and your family's health after the birth. The confidence you develop can build self-reliance and increased skill in ensuring good health for your growing baby, as well as for yourself and your whole family.

It's well worth becoming a strong guardian of your family's health. As a practical matter you will often be the one who makes the initial decision that a certain illness needs to be treated by a health professional rather than in the home. Your partner may also share and carry out this role.

With practice, you can exchange your old habit of blindly relying on outside medical authority for a beneficial new role: you can learn to place the primary reliance for family health measures on yourselves. Authorities will then serve you in partnership as advisors and sources of information, rather than in the role of infallible superhumans. (Remember that your old attitudes may not be easy to change.)

Whatever your choice about the role you want to take in childbearing, it should make you comfortable rather than anxious, because your emotions are vitally important to your well-being and that of your baby. At Maternity Center Association's Childbearing Center, for example, if either a mother or her family members seem nervous about being enrolled, we encourage that family to seek care where they can be more at ease, and we assist them in doing so.

Unfortunately, some of you reading this book may not have a full range of options. If such is the case and you want a different approach, you might discuss your desires with the available provider(s) and also make requests directly to hospital administrators or boards of directors. Others among you may not learn of the alternatives until you enroll in prenatal classes and talk to other expectant couples. You may then realize that you are not happy with your current care-provider but may be fearful of making a change.

7

The best approach in such a situation may well be to talk over your uneasiness with that provider. Most care-providers would want you to be where you are most comfortable. Remember, they are there to care for you. Your feelings are central. You are purchasing an important service and should feel completely satisfied with it.

Still others among you may feel strongly that you *do* want an authority to direct you, or perhaps that you do want the conventional separation from your infant in the hospital. If you're a busy mother of small children, you may well look forward to a rest in the hospital and to being taken care of yourself for a change. (However, if you are extremely exhausted from housework and child care, you should have some rest and relief *during* your pregnancy—right now—and not have to wait for the birth to get a respite.)

Some readers' decisions regarding care may be influenced by other family members and the desire to please. Again, we remind you that you and your feelings are central. At the Childbearing Center, we learned at one time that some of our young families were not telling their own parents of their enrollment because they thought their parents would be strongly critical. So we offered our clients the opportunity to bring their parents along to see for themselves and to talk with us—a "grandparents' night."

It was wonderful to see those fears being reduced. We also heard some of the expectant grandmothers recount the unhappiness they had felt with their own long-ago childbirth experiences. Of course, most had given birth when amnesics and general anesthesia were in vogue.

Birth situations in which the mother's and the family's feelings are given low priority remain with us still. The following anecdote describes the struggles of a woman physician with her own emotions regarding birth.

As a medical student, intern, and resident, Pat Solomon Rodriguez had felt that her reaction to taking part in hospital childbirth was different from her colleagues', who retained an aloof, detached, impassive attitude when working with women in labor and birth. In contrast, Dr. Rodriguez experienced intense emotions of elation, sympathy, and tenderness toward the mother and infant all during labor and delivery. But she feared that these feelings reflected a serious professional shortcoming in herself. An M.D. specializing in pediatrics, she struggled to control such feelings and expected to get over them in time.

It was with the birth of her first child, Kira, that her views began to change. Dr. Rodriguez chose a fellow physician for her childbearing care, a female obstetrician widely respected as forward-looking and dedicated to women's interests.

Dr. Rodriguez accordingly had her first labor and childbirth at a large city hospital where her obstetrician was on the staff. The hospital had recently introduced the use of certified nurse-midwives working with the obstetricians in its maternity care.

"A nurse-midwife was with me all through my first labor, and I liked her special caring and warmth," Dr. Rodriguez says. But in spite of this, the standard hospital routine for rather conventional birth was very much in evidence. "The baby was whisked away just after I'd had only the briefest chance to hold her."

The hospital followed the pattern for conventional hospital childbirth in other ways, including birth in a labor and delivery area outfitted essentially as a surgical operating facility, and conventional positioning for birth (lying on the back with legs up in stirrups). But what Dr. Rodriguez noticed most of all was the relative unresponsiveness of those attending the birth. She had learned Lamaze breathing and exercises and needed no anesthetics during labor. As a result, she was acutely alert and even elated all through her labor and delivery. But some of the staff attending her talked among themselves as if she were unconscious, rather than wide awake and concentrating on an enormously important and exciting task.

In addition, the rooming-in service provided by the hospital "really wasn't rooming-in at all," Dr. Rodriguez says. The baby was left with her mother just for feeding rather than for any length of time.

In many ways the experience left her dissatisfied. It made her think that perhaps her own natural reactions while attending birth as a physician might not be as wrong as she'd imagined.

Her dissatisfaction with that first experience made Dr. Rodriguez curious about the Childbearing Center. She heard of the Center early in her second pregnancy, and she became increasingly pleased with it the more she learned. Her husband, Julio, also liked the idea of having their baby there. Years before, his mother had been assisted during his own birth at home through the former field nurse-midwifery service of the Maternity Center Association.

One thing about the Center appealed to Dr. Rodriguez especially: the thoroughness with which it served all the needs, emotional as well as physical, of the childbearing family. Other features she strongly approved of included its homelike nature in actual functioning as well as appearance, combined with rigorous professional safeguards and prompt hospital backup if needed. She determined that, for her, the risk associated with possible transfer to a hospital during labor or birth was outweighed by a number of factors. These included

- the careful continuous health screening of all enrolled women,
- the care by nurse-midwives, centered on prevention and early detection of problems,

- the chosen obstetrical backup at the receiving hospital, and
- the emergency equipment available in the center.

She approved also of its arrangements for letting others share in the experience of the birth, among them adult family members, other children, and close friends. Dr. Rodriguez and her husband enrolled in the Childbearing Center, including the prenatal classes required for those families electing to use the program, for their second pregnancy and birth. Their satisfaction with that experience led them to return later for their third pregnancy and birth.

Evaluate the Risks of Advanced Technology and Birth in a Hospital

There's one very important point to keep in mind when you're just starting out in the decision-making process:

> *Do not assume that birth in a hospital (or in any other setting) is risk-free. Also, do not assume that advanced technologies such as amniocentesis, ultrasound scans, and electronic fetal monitoring pose few or no risks of their own. All options have both benefits and risks. Find out about the risks inherent in any facet of the new technology, and take such risks into account when selecting the option which is best for you in your circumstances.*

It is easy to assume that hospital settings and advanced technologies are safest. They do tend to be the alternatives least questioned by medical specialists. But any intervention carries its own risk, even if small. You should run these risks only if they're justified.

Understand How You Can Influence the Choices That Are Available

As you start out in your own childbearing experience, it's also important for you to know that you and other expectant parents can play a decisive part in having better, more responsive ways of childbirth made available. The fact is that interested expectant parents like yourselves often have been crucially responsible for winning needed reforms.

Suppose you discover that a certain alternative you very much want, such as rooming-in, is not offered in your community. You might find it worthwhile to join with others to work toward provision of that service.

Knowing that you can be actively involved in bringing about change is important. Options that are available in a great many places today were made possible in large part by the efforts of childbearing families of earlier years. These families often worked to ensure that alternatives they couldn't have themselves would be available to younger persons—including their own sons and daughters. You might share such an interest yourself.

Childbirth education classes, rooming-in, and alternative birth environments were all made possible by consumer demand and, in the case of the Maternity Center Association, consumer response. MCA is a voluntary health agency. Its board consists of consumers working with professional advisory groups. Since its founding in 1918, MCA has been responsible for initiating prenatal care, prenatal parent education, prepared childbirth, nurse-midwifery education, and freestanding birth centers in the U.S. It has helped other consumer groups and families make their voices heard.

As another example, the La Leche League has become famous worldwide for its influence in reviving the practice of feeding babies at breast instead of with formulas. Through the League, mothers help teach and encourage others to breastfeed. The organization traces its origin to a conversation at a picnic in 1956 between Marion Thompson and Mary White, who went on to found the League. La Leche has since grown to include some 4,000 chapters in 50 countries, with 12,000 women serving as volunteer group leaders.

Once You Begin to Make Decisions

This book is intended to help you with every aspect of childbearing, from relieving minor discomforts to questions of life and death. It attempts to acquaint you with all the ways in which you can benefit yourself and your unborn baby by understanding and choosing wisely from the range of options open to you.

With the advice given here, you will be better able to decide what you need to do to prepare actively for birth, and how you'll feed your baby, get members of your family ready for the baby's arrival, and prepare your home and yourself for the new family member.

In helping with all your momentous decisions about labor and birth, we try to be as evenhanded as possible in acquainting you with all the major alternatives so that you can choose the way *you think best fits you* for normal childbearing. And should you run into complications or abnormalities, you'll have other decisions to make, for which we also have some suggestions.

One last reminder: Relish the freedom you have to make informed, conscious, deliberate choices. Know about the variety of options open to you. You *will* be choosing among them, either deliberately or by default. Why not enjoy the fulfillment of making these decisions yourself?

2

꙰ꙮꙬꙮ꙰

First Decisions

Now let's build on your philosophy about childbearing by filling in what gaps there may be in your knowledge, so that you can become better able to make sound decisions for yourself, your baby, and your family. Be sure also to draw on further sources of help by attending prenatal classes, talking with other parents and expectant parents, and reading widely while you compare your prior impressions with your own pregnancy experience.

As you progress through your pregnancy and learn more about the incomparable design of your body and its processes in supporting your growing baby, you will feel a growing sense of fascination. The more you know, the more miraculous you will find pregnancy.

Knowing what is involved in your own pregnancy can help make it an even more meaningful and satisfying experience. Even the occasional discomforts, fears, disappointments, and times of distress can become productive challenges. You can rise to these with increased capability, confidence, and strength once you learn why they develop and understand how you can cope with them.

How Do You Know You're Pregnant?

How you choose to confirm your pregnancy is one of your important early decisions.

Observing Signs in Your Body

Knowing pregnancy is possible, some women enjoy the anticipation of waiting for their bodies to tell them they have conceived. A few sense emotionally that they're pregnant right from the start. Physically, a missed menstrual period is a time-honored sign of pregnancy. ("Amenorrhea" is the term you may hear used for this condition.) You can watch for further signs, too, like these.

- You might notice changes in your breasts in the early weeks. Your breasts may tingle. The reddish circles around your nipples—the areolae—may darken, and the tiny bumps on them called Montgomery's tubercles may become more prominent. Also, the blood vessels within your breasts will slowly become more visible through the skin.
- You might begin to notice that you feel more tired at times, or drowsier than usual, reflecting your body's natural demand for more rest.
- You could start getting sudden cravings for certain foods as your body starts to nourish the growing embryo.
- You may feel a need to urinate more often than before, when the early growth of your uterus deep in your abdomen begins to crowd your bladder.
- You may also begin to dislike some of your favorite foods, you may feel nauseous or actually experience vomiting. This happens to perhaps a third or a half of expectant mothers in the first few months of pregnancy (and is traditionally though mistakenly called morning sickness).
- You may notice changes in your sexual desires. Some women find they enjoy intercourse more during pregnancy, whereas others come to dislike coitus while pregnant. Openness and consideration between partners can effectively deal with either possibility.

Pregnancy Tests

Because of the importance of beginning prenatal care early, you may be interested in being tested for pregnancy after you have missed a period. Understand, though, that you certainly do not need a test if you and your care-giver decide it's satisfactory for you to let the natural signs appear over time.

However, tests may have practical advantages in certain situations.

- *Seeing if you're pregnant before missing a period:* Even before you've missed a period, you could confirm whether you're pregnant or not through one fairly simple test.
- *Seeing if you're pregnant when a missed period could have some other cause:* Pregnancy tests might be helpful to you because periods can be late or missed for reasons other than pregnancy—such as illness, intensive sports exertion, or other unusual stress in your life.
- *Seeing if you're pregnant even though you have discharge resembling periods:* A few women have what may appear to be menstrual periods in the early months of pregnancy, though typically with decreased flow and of shorter duration than is customary for them.

Pregnancy Tests: Key Features

Test Type	Earliest Use	Main Advantage	Main Disadvantage
Home-use tests, urine	6–7 weeks after last period began	Self-administered	Highly reliable only if positive
Home-use tests, new type	10–14 days after conception	Early; self-administered	May not be highly reliable even if positive
Laboratory tests, urine	6–7 weeks after last period began	More reliable than home-use tests	Inconvenience of going to laboratory or clinic
Blood test	7–10 days after conception	Highly reliable	Limited availability; often expensive

Home-use pregnancy tests: Several brands of home-use pregnancy tests have been available without prescription since the late 1970s. To carry out one of these tests, you use a sample of your urine. A positive finding of pregnancy is thought to have a high probability of accuracy. A negative result ("not pregnant") with one of these tests, though, may be wrong perhaps 20 percent of the time. As a result, you should not rely on a negative finding with a home test.

Two weeks after you've missed your period is the earliest time usually recommended for making one of these urine-based tests (that is, not earlier than six weeks from the first day of your last menstrual period). If you have an irregular menstrual cycle, you should wait until three weeks after you've missed your period (rather than two weeks) to carry out a home-use test. The directions may suggest using the test as early as six to ten days after your first missed period, but this is generally too early to be accurate.

Some brands of these home pregnancy tests claim that they can be used far earlier—as early as ten days after conception. Pharmacists comment that these tests are reasonably accurate in the case of positive results, especially if used two weeks or more after conception. One test kit of this type provides for making two tests in order to ensure higher reliability.

What the tests analyze is the presence of a hormone called human chorionic gonadotrophin (HCG). It is found in the urine of pregnant women, in amounts that slowly increase as pregnancy advances, with a peak around the third month. Taking a urine test too early may yield erroneous results because the HCG concentration might not be detectable yet.

Laboratory tests with urine: Two types of laboratory tests using urine are widely available for determining pregnancy. As with the home-use tests, both types analyze for the presence of the hormone HCG. For reliable results, neither type should be used any earlier than two weeks after you've missed your period.

One type is quite similar to the home-use test, but it may be more dependable because it's done under laboratory conditions. These tests are sometimes called the immunologic type, inasmuch as they involve a reaction between HCG and certain antibodies with which they are placed in contact.

The other types of laboratory urine test, used much less often, involves injection of some sample urine into a laboratory animal. Originally a rabbit was used, and therefore the test was often called the rabbit test.

The cost of a laboratory urine test may be about the same as a home-use test kit, particularly if you go to a clinic such as Planned Parenthood or other women's facility. And if laboratory testing results appear inconclusive for any reason, a repeat test is sometimes made free of charge.

Blood tests: As early as seven to ten days after conception (and thus even before a missed menstrual period), a blood sample can be tested for pregnancy. This test is said to be highly reliable for positive results. You might therefore consider it if you want to be especially sure of the results, or want a more conclusive second test.

Because special equipment is used for the blood test, it is usually available only through larger medical centers or laboratories, and it is more expensive than the urine laboratory tests. The level of HCG in the blood is evaluated through radioreceptor assay (RRA); the blood sample is mixed with radioactive substances. Radioimmuno assay (RIA) is a similar blood test for pregnancy. It is often more expensive than the RRA test, but is considered more reliable in indicating pregnancy as early as a week after conception. These tests are advisable if you might be contemplating x-ray examinations or surgery for some other condition and could be pregnant at the time.

The progesterone test: Another type of pregnancy test is occasionally used by physicians. The woman is prescribed progesterone, one of the hormones of pregnancy, for several days in a row—usually because her period is late. If she is not pregnant, menstruation will begin two to seven days after she stops taking the progesterone. However, recent evidence indicates that progesterone has adverse effects on female fetuses, resulting in an increased likelihood of developing genital cancers as they mature. *We do not recommend this test.*

Physical examination: Your care-giver can also determine that conception has occurred by examining your genitalia. The cervix, or mouth of the womb, softens soon after conception and the vaginal mucosa (mucous membrane) becomes congested and bluish in color. Internal examination will reveal changes in uterine size, even though the uterus is not palpable abdominally until about the twelfth week of pregnancy.

Estimating the Date of Your Baby's Birth

At this point, you can figure out your baby's probable birth date just as well as any obstetrical specialist. In fact, figuring it out depends on information only you can give. And it's easy.

Pregnancies, from conception to the spontaneous beginning of labor, vary in length with the average being 266 days. In standard professional practice, the expected date of birth is calculated to be 280 days (40 weeks) after the first day of your last menstrual period. ("EDC" identifies that date on your medical records; it stands for the old-fashioned term "expected date of confinement.") This calculation assumes that the ovulation resulting in your pregnancy occurred about halfway between your menstrual periods: the 266-day average plus 14 days (counting back to ovulation) gives 280 days, or 40 weeks. The week of pregnancy you are in is counted on this 40-week basis, starting from the first day of your last menstrual period.

You can estimate your EDC by adding 7 days to the date on which your last menstrual period began; then count back three months to get your EDC. (Counting back gives the same answer as counting forward nine months, but it's simpler.) For example, suppose that your last menstrual period began on August 1. Adding 7 days to that gives August 8. Counting back three months gives EDC of May 8. If your regular menstrual cycle is longer than 28 days, make a further, final adjustment: add to the EDC the difference between your cycle and 28 days (if your cycle is 30 days, add 2 to the May 8 date, to give an EDC of May 10).

If you are uncertain about the date of your last menstrual period or have a very irregular cycle, your baby's due date might also be estimated in other ways, such as by noting the first occasion on which the fetal heartbeat can be heard. This exciting event usually takes place when the fetus is 18 to 20 weeks old, if a stethoscope is used, or when it is 12 weeks old if a hand-held ultrasound apparatus is used. This method estimates fetal age with an accuracy of about two weeks.

You should consider one further method only if you have an essential reason for estimating the EDC accurately, because its possible risks for your unborn baby are as yet not fully known. The method involves making an ultrasound scan, which provides pictorial images of the fetus in the uterus. The eighth week of pregnancy is about the earliest that useful results can be obtained. A scan specialist should be able to estimate the age of the fetus to an accuracy of about a week.

You might have to go to a hospital for a scan, but some physicians have the equipment in their offices. A scan involves what amounts to an office visit and only the minimal discomfort associated with a full bladder. (You will be asked to drink several glasses of water so that the full bladder pushes the uterus up out of the pelvis, so it can be better visualized.) Scans can be quite expensive.

Scans, the hand-held apparatus, and external electronic fetal monitors all operate by projecting sound waves and interpreting their reflection, as described in Chapter 6.

If You're Over 35 and Having Your First Baby

Most American women do have their first children while still in their twenties; the average age of new mothers is around 24. However, increasing numbers of women today first become mothers at ages past

30, and up to 40 or even 45. As you might expect, this stems from the increased numbers of women who concentrate on careers in their twenties and thirties. (In the past such women over 35 were referred to as elderly primigravidas, and considered to have special problems because of their age.) These pregnancies of healthy women over 35 who had borne children at young ages were considered to be more predictable because of the evidence of past childbearing experience. However, the conditions which occur with greater frequency as age increases affect all childbearing women, not only those having a first baby.

A recent study by the National Center for Health Statistics found that the number of first births to American women in their thirties more than doubled during the decade of the 1970s. Birth-certificate data showed that there were more than 115,000 such mothers in 1979, as against 54,108 in 1970. Much of the increase came among women with more education, incidentally. Of the first-time mothers in the study's 30-to-34 age group, only 28 percent of those who gave birth in 1970 had finished four years of college, compared to nearly 50 percent who had done so among those giving birth in 1979.

Certain special information can be helpful if you're having your first baby and are over the age of 35. Probably most important *from the standard of health, having your first child this late very probably will result in a completely normal baby and a thoroughly normal and satisfying pregnancy and birth experience.* That's especially true if you are generally healthy and fit and are eager to carry out thorough prenatal care and proper nutrition. You and the baby may even realize some unusual advantages.

By no means should you be overly troubled by widespread medical opinions, lingering from earlier days, that childless women in or past their mid-thirties necessarily run large risks of having difficult births or defective babies with their first pregnancy. However, you should know that some risks to the baby and mother do tend to be higher with mothers over age 35 (or even 30) than with younger mothers. Precautions against those risks can prove largely effective.

Down Syndrome

With increasing maternal age, the frequency of births of infants with Down syndrome (formerly called Mongolism) increases. Down syndrome is characterized by marked mental retardation and a unique physical appearance. Children born with this syndrome usually have difficult health problems and have special social, emotional, and educational needs.

Down syndrome results from a genetic defect in the twenty-first chromosome in the egg cell. It is progressively more likely to occur as a woman gets older. For mothers of differing age levels, the incidence of the syndrome is approximately as follows:

45 years and above: about 1 in 40 pregnancies

40 to 45, about 1 in 100

35 to 40, about 1 in 400

30 to 35, about 1 in 900

20 to 30, about 1 in 2,000

Almost certain diagnosis of Down syndrome can be obtained through a test procedure called amniocentesis. If carried out, it should be done in about the fourteenth through sixteenth week of pregnancy. It provides results some two to three weeks later. Approximately one hundred other types of rarer birth defects can also be revealed by this technique.

Some families who learn through the test that their fetus has Down syndrome may consider terminating the pregnancy.

Amniocentesis poses some slight risks: infection, hemorrhage, and perhaps miscarriage. By slight, we mean less than about 1 chance in 200 to 500. Amniocentesis entails a medical office visit and minor discomfort for the mother. It is done by a specialist and costs several hundred dollars.

An expectant couple over age 35 or 40 might weigh various factors in reaching a decision concerning possible Down syndrome. If they absolutely would not consider abortion, they should hope for the best and reject amniocentesis. If they have strong reservations about abortion and very much want to avoid any chance of a miscarriage, they might also reject amniocentesis. On the other hand, an older couple who believes it vitally important to avoid having a Down syndrome baby might decide to go ahead with amniocentesis. In any event, you should be guided in any such decision by competent professional authorities.

Complications in Childbirth

In past eras pregnant women over age 35 or 40 tended to have somewhat higher incidence of complications in childbirth itself, with a related higher incidence of delivery by cesarean section. Older mothers who had borne large numbers of children, closely spaced, did indeed have more complications. But childbirth professionals around the country report that today's older mothers have had fewer children than their earlier counterparts. In addition, these mothers typically make sure they have high-quality prenatal care.

Family Considerations

Some couples in their forties have voiced concerns of another kind. In radio broadcasts and public-forum programs in which we have taken part, about half the questions came from men in their forties asking how to cope with having a first baby and at the same time cope with the aging of their parents, the grandparents of the unborn child. As this concern suggests, there may be family and social considerations other than the possible physical risks in later parenting.

The risks you might run in having a first baby when you're over 35 or 40 should not keep you from appreciating the many advantages that more mature parenthood can bring. For example, later parenting can allow for advanced career progress for both mother and father by the time their parenting begins. It can mean a more settled life for a couple, especially deep interest in a new baby, and greater freedom from distractions and insecurities than in earlier years. On the other hand, a high level of energy is necessary to care for young children, and older couples might find parenting more tiring.

It's almost impossible to make a conclusive case for childbearing earlier or later in prime adult years. But the advantages that can be realized by later parenting couples are certainly attractive.

Choosing a "Family"

How bizarre, you may think—one cannot choose one's own family! Of course you're right. You can't choose your relatives (or "consanguinal kin," as anthropologists term those related to you by blood line). But those persons you choose to support you with affection, knowledge, and care during your pregnancy and birth experience should be people who inspire in you positive feelings of family, whether they are actually related or not.

You may decide to have your sister, mother, aunt, or cousin with you (probably in addition to the baby's father). Or you may decide on a close friend. At our childbearing center, we encourage mothers to select their closest kin (even if those individuals are fictive kin) because we know that peace of mind is an important factor during pregnancy, in labor, and throughout the early days of parenthood.

3

～〜〜〜

Early Pregnancy: The First Trimester

Pregnancy Begins

Your baby begins as a ripening egg cell (the largest human cell, about the size of a dot over an "i" and just barely visible to the naked eye). To understand precisely what happens to that cell, look at Figure 3.1 to see which organs carry out each step.

That egg cell ripens in the ovary (number 1 in the diagram on page 24) when triggered to do so by a hormone produced by the pituitary gland at the base of the brain. The ovary then secretes the hormone estrogen into the bloodstream, blocking the pituitary from making more egg-ripening hormone and at the same time stimulating the lining of the uterus to thicken (in readiness for a fertilized egg). The egg is then released from a special bulge, or follicle, on the ovary's surface. Fringes of tissue called fimbria (3) at the open end of the fallopian tube "catch" the ripe egg cell and start it traveling through the tube toward the uterus, or womb (2).

All figures in this chapter are reprinted by permission of Maternity Center Association from the *Birth Atlas* and *A Baby Is Born: The Picture Story of Everyman's Beginning,* sculptures by Dr. Robert L. Dickinson and Abram Belskie, drawings by Frank Robinson, copyright © by Maternity Center Association 1940, 1945, 1957, 1960, 1964, 1966, 1968, 1970, 1973, 1974, 1975, 1977, 1978. All rights reserved. Additional illustrations from these works appear in Chapters 5 (Figure 5.2), 7, 8, and 13.

That follicle on the ovary becomes the corpus luteum and begins to make progesterone, which prepares the uterus for receiving a fertilized egg—and, if the egg *is* fertilized, the corpus luteum continues to make progesterone all through pregnancy, thereby suppressing the menstrual cycle. But if the egg is not fertilized, within several days the follicle closes up and progesterone output declines sharply. As a result, the lining of the uterus with its rich blood supply sloughs away, and the woman has a menstrual period.

Figure 3.1 also shows the protective bones surrounding the internal organs: in front, the pubic bone (4); in back, the sacrum (5) and the coccyx (6); and on both sides, the hipbones (not pictured).

The bladder (7) is usually crowded by the enlarging uterus, resulting in more frequent urination; the bladder outlet is the urethra (8). Shown also are the lower end of the uterus, called the cervix (9), opening into the upper end of the vagina (10), or birth canal. In addition, you can see the lower bowel (11); the rectum, or collecting point (12);

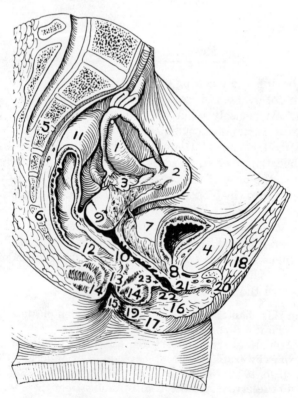

Numbered diagram for Figure 3.1.

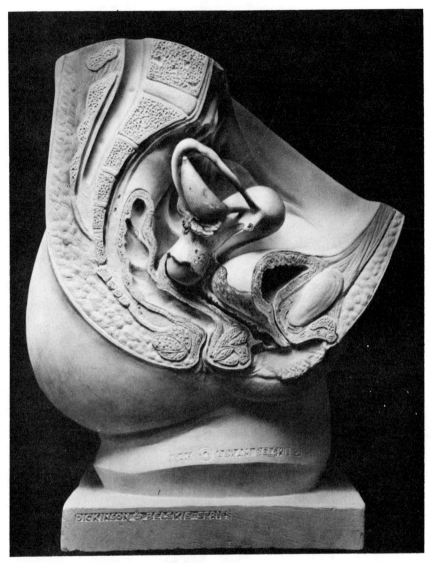

Figure 3.1. The woman's reproductive organs

and the anal canal (13), with the sphincter muscles (14), which close the anus (15), the actual opening for defecation.

External organs and structures include the labia minora (16) and labia majora (17), extending down from the mons veneris (18) to the perineum (19); and the clitoris (20), urethral outlet (21), vaginal outlet (22), and hymen (23).

The man's organs involved in fertilizing the egg are illustrated in Figure 3.2. The one sperm cell that fertilizes the egg is produced, along with millions of other sperm cells, in the hundreds of feet of microscopic tubules within one of the two testes (1) and (2) in the scrotum (3). The sperm then are shifted to a larger tube coiled behind each testis, the epididymis (4); next the sperm travel through the vas deferens, the sperm duct (5), for storage in the enlarged end of the duct, the ampulla (6).

In sexual excitement, the penis (7) becomes erect, the outlet from the bladder (8) is closed, and sperm move out of the ampulla into the ejaculatory duct (11). Secretions from the Cowper's glands (9), each seminal vesicle (12), and the prostate gland (13) mix with the sperm. In orgasm, about a spoonful of this seminal fluid, containing millions of tiny sperm cells, is ejaculated through the end of the urethra (10) into the vagina. Each sperm cell consists of a small oval-shaped head containing 23 chromosomes, and a long whiplike tail that propels the cell and is absorbed during fertilization.

Fertilization occurs as shown in Figure 3.3, which presents a frontal cross-sectional view of the uterus, attached fallopian tubes, or oviducts,

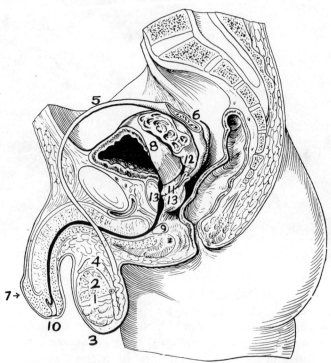

Numbered diagram for Figure 3.2.

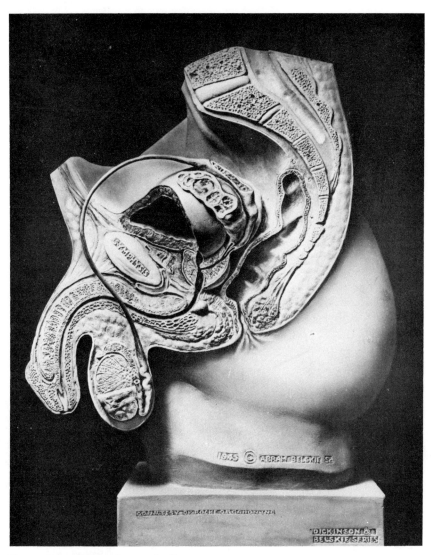

Figure 3.2. The man's reproductive organs

on each side, and the ovaries. Near the outer end of the tube on the left is pictured a ripe egg cell surrounded by long-tailed sperm (for visibility, egg and sperm are depicted greatly magnified). The mobile sperm have been drawn along from the vagina, through the cervix, into the uterus, and along the oviduct to the egg. Except in the case of multiple births, only one sperm penetrates the egg nucleus, in effect

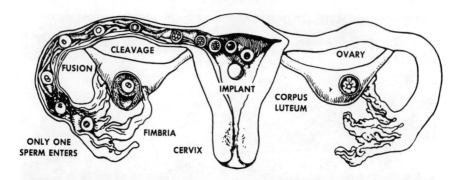

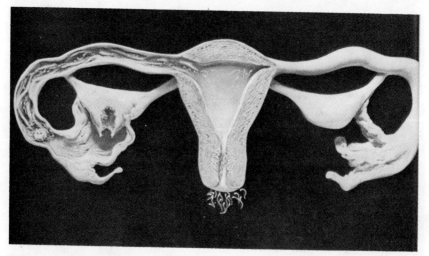

Figure 3.3. Fertilization

closing the egg to all other sperm. The twenty-three chromosomes of the egg cell and the sperm cell combine to comprise the forty-six chromosomes found in each body cell of the human species. The fertilized egg begins the process of division into two, four, and eight cells, and on and on into the development of a complete human being.

The Fourth and Sixth Weeks

Just about the time a pregnant woman notices that her period has failed to develop, some four weeks after her last period, the unborn baby is about the size of a small button, as shown at the top in Figure 3.4. In the photograph, the baby appears as the whitish dot to the right of center in the fundus, the upper part of the uterus (smaller

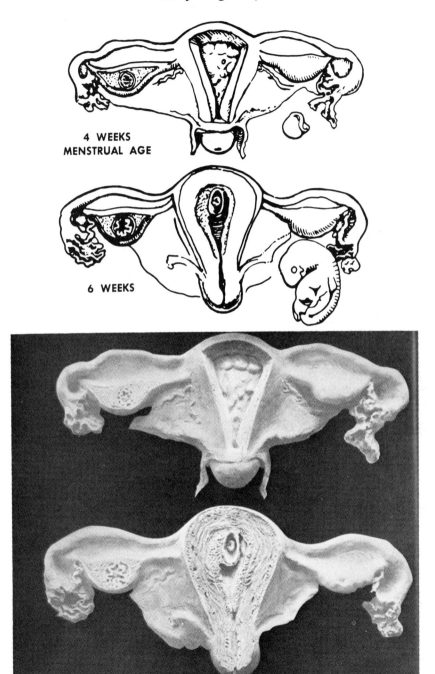

4 WEEKS
MENSTRUAL AGE

6 WEEKS

Figure 3.4. Fourth and sixth weeks of pregnancy

and below the three rounded bumps at the top). The baby (now called an embryo) has settled into the soft uterine lining and is growing very rapidly. (The star-shaped structure at the far left on the ovary is the corpus luteum.)

About two weeks later, after the sixth week of pregnancy, the embryo has developed as pictured in the upper illustrations and will soon be called a fetus. The embryo floats, cushioned and insulated in fluid, within the double-walled membrane called the amniotic sac, usually near the top of the uterus. The baby's heart has begun to beat, but too quietly to be heard. The uterine wall has greatly thickened, and between it and the sac the placenta is developing (shown as the spongy structure to the left of the sac). The placenta is the remarkable temporary structure through which food and oxygen are filtered from the mother's bloodstream and waste products are removed. Tiny blood vessels from the baby's circulatory system contact the mother's blood to exchange materials through the vessel walls. There is no actual exchange of circulating blood between the mother and the fetus. However, harmful substances as well as essential nutriments can pass through the placenta from the mother to the baby.

Around the time of the second missed period (or earlier), the internal genitalia will reflect changes. As evident in a pelvic examination, the cervix will have softened from its usual firmness (like the tip of the nose) to feel more like lips (such softening is termed Goodell's sign). The color of the vaginal walls and cervix will also have changed, from pink to a more bluish hue (Chadwick's sign).

The Tenth Week

By the tenth week, the developing fetus has begun to look like a baby, with clearly recognizable legs, arms, head, and trunk, as shown in Figure 3.5. It is about 2 or 2½ inches long (5 or 6 centimeters). The placenta has become much larger, and the walls of the uterus have grown thicker still.

The movements of the unborn baby cannot yet be felt by the mother. The enlarging uterus hasn't begun to push out the abdomen noticeably, but it can be palpated, or felt from the outside, between the hands of an examining nurse-midwife or physician.

Changes in Your Emotions

Pregnancy marks a major change in the lives of a couple. The woman consequently experiences powerful changes in her emotions, along

FROM REAR

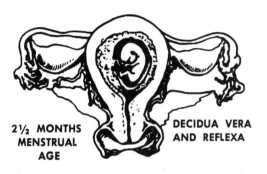

2 ½ MONTHS
MENSTRUAL
AGE

DECIDUA VERA
AND REFLEXA

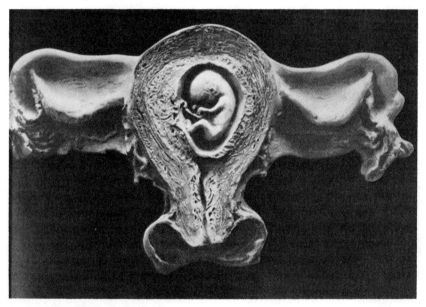

Figure 3.5. Tenth week of pregnancy

with the physical developments of early pregnancy. Hormonal changes in her system add to these shifts in emotion. The expectant father may feel similar emotions.

You can expect that your feelings in pregnancy will often be conflicting ones. Among the positive emotions can be an unlifting sense of fulfillment, a feeling of great creative powers and vitality, passionate affection, and keen anticipation and excitement. Negative emotions, on the other hand, can include concern about your ability to cope with parenthood and its responsibilities, worry over the coming loss of independence, fear of losing some of the love and closeness of your partner, and anxiety about the "ordeal" of pregnancy, labor, and birth.

Mood swings are common. Most pregnant women laugh and cry more easily than before they conceived. To reinforce your positive feelings, try taking actions like the following ones.

Give positive emotions free play: Take advantage of the natural lift that comes with pregnancy. Enjoy that deep sense of fulfillment; your feeling of having vast creative powers and vitality flow through you unchecked. Don't hold back on expressing impulses of passionate affection, especially to your partner. When you feel a rapturous glow of anticipation and excitement, savor it.

Make a conscious effort to stir up these positive feelings whenever negative ones start bothering you.

Take special care of yourself: Put in extra time to care for your appearance, health, and comfort. Keeping attractive and fit will help dispel any worries about not looking as appealing as you did before. And making sure you have enough rest and nourishment helps guard against low spirits and annoyance.

Show special love for your partner: You can draw on the heightened affection often felt in pregnancy to be especially warm and loving with your partner. If you're having a normal, low-risk pregnancy, you can engage in intercourse all through pregnancy without harm to yourself or the baby.

Like many couples, you may find sexual attraction heightened during pregnancy. If you have greater sexual appetite than usual, by all means feel free to convey this special love for your partner with more intercourse than usual. As your uterus grows, your partner may not want to rest his weight on you. To make this easier, many couples use different positions in intercourse. For example, a favored position to avoid strain in the weeks just before labor is with the woman lying on her side and the man behind her penetrating vaginally from the rear.

However, decreased interest in sex when pregnant is also perfectly normal. If pregnancy has lowered your interest in intercourse, show special love for your partner in as many other ways as possible. Explain to him that your lack of libido in no way affects your deep love for him. You can satisfy him sexually without intercourse, in ways you probably employed in lovemaking before the pregnancy occurred, such as petting to orgasm.

Expressing special love in these ways helps generate the positive emotions of pregnancy both in yourself and in your partner, with mutually reinforcing effects.

Talk in honest intimacy with your partner: Talking to your partner with utter honesty about your most intimate feelings can be one of your most effective ways of feeling positive about having a baby. Be frank in discussing things that trouble you about your pregnancy, and other things that delight you. Open communication is often easier when the feelings of both expectant parents are closer to the surface.

In case you haven't already made it a habit to have such times of honest, intimate talk, here's how you might begin.

Decide on a First Topic: To start, pick one topic you want to talk about. Try to choose something that really concerns you but that you think won't be too unsettling to your partner. For instance, you might start with worries about how you'll be tied down looking after the baby and not as independent as you had been before. However, go ahead on a possibly alarming topic—your fears over having a baby with a serious birth defect, perhaps—if you feel you really have to talk about it first.

Start Talking on a Quiet, Untroubled Occasion: Pick a private time when neither of you feels pressed to do something else. Then, tell your partner that you want to talk over something very honestly and closely. A kiss or a hug or holding hands may help set an atmosphere of closeness. Then say very honestly what you feel, and ask what he honestly feels.

Talk Only About the One Topic: Once you both have talked out your feelings about the topic you've brought up, be ready to stop there. It's very likely that you will have relieved your troubled feelings and will have cleared away similar feelings for your partner. Leave other concerns for later. Having started honest, intimate communication will make it all the easier the next time.

Find other women to talk with: Talking over your feelings and thoughts with other women who are also pregnant or who have recently given birth can help strengthen your positive emotions about pregnancy. You might choose friends or relatives to talk with warmly and openly. But if no friends or relatives would be quite right for this, you can be almost certain to find others who are especially helpful to talk with through a prenatal class or self-help group. (The Appendices give information on locating these.)

Seek full answers to your health concerns from sources you trust: Not knowing what's happening to you or what you should do in pregnancy can undercut your positive emotions. Head off any negative feelings that might be caused by ignorance by seeking answers to vexing questions from sources you trust, such as your care-givers. Teachers of prenatal classes can also help.

Take prenatal classes with your partner: Taking prenatal classes with your partner can help to foster a positive attitude. Many classes today provide programs for the expectant mother and father together. Having your partner prepare with you for an active support role throughout pregnancy, labor, and birth is viewed as very important by the sponsors of these classes. So important do they consider such a support role that they urge the woman to have a close woman friend or relative attend with her if the father for some reason cannot.

You and your partner can benefit in a number of ways from going to prenatal classes together—acquiring knowledge and understanding, and developing important skills to use together in prenatal exercises and in giving birth to your child. Your closeness to each other should be increased by attending classes together, and you'll both be helped by talking with other expectant couples. Childbirth educators can also direct you to books such as this one.

Should you and your partner take these actions and still find yourselves troubled by negative emotions, seek out one additional source of help: professional counseling or therapy. Qualified counselors can be recommended by the nurse-midwife, physician, or other practitioner you have chosen for guidance through pregnancy and birth. Therapy can help relieve the sharp emotional stress that expecting a child imposes on some individuals and couples. But for most expectant parents, the suggestions here are more than enough to help you feel really good about having a baby.

4

Weight Gain and Nutrition

Your choices about the kinds and amounts of foods to eat during pregnancy are especially important. Only by eating properly can you provide all the nutrients that are essential for your unborn baby and for your own health. You'll need to make sound decisions in two main areas for adequate nutrition:

- gaining enough weight.
- eating the right foods.

> *Reject the idea that the fetus will automatically get all it needs from your own system.*

Though widespread, that idea is wrong—a myth, an "old wives' tale."

Remember this instead: Only those foods actually present in your bloodstream every day readily reach your unborn baby. The baby can suffer damage from poor nutrition if you are badly undernourished.

Gain Enough Weight

Be sure to gain enough weight to safeguard good health for you and your baby. Resist limiting your weight for reasons like these:

- A prepregnancy habit of holding your weight down by dieting or skipping meals.

- Memories of past practice of physicians to rigidly limit weight gain of pregnant women. So widespread was this practice that in 1972, 60 to 70 percent of expectant mothers were prescribed diuretics, or "water pills," to trim excess weight.[1] (The U.S. Food and Drug Administration today warns expectant mothers not to take diuretics, because they can be hazardous in pregnancy.)

Your weight gain in pregnancy as currently recommended by various authorities may range from 20 to 40 pounds (and more, with twins or other multiple-birth pregnancies).

Many experts emphasize smaller ranges. For example, here is the recommendation made jointly by the American College of Obstetricians and Gynecologists and the American Academy of Pediatrics[2]:

> Universal agreement has never been achieved on how much weight should be gained in pregnancy. More important than total weight gain is the pattern of weight gain. Maximal gain occurs during the second trimester, although from a practical point of view the rate of gain is essentially linear after the tenth gestational week, averaging about 0.4 kg/week. The usual average weight gain, therefore, is 10–12 kg (22–27 lb).

That "0.4 kg/week" comes to about nine-tenths of a pound, or 14 ounces per week on the average.

Two more actions are strongly recommended in the same report:

1. It is essential to get expert help if you have *not* gained at least 9 to 11 pounds by midpregnancy (about the twentieth week).
2. It is important for all expectant mothers, and especially those who are obese, *not* to diet in order to lose weight during pregnancy or while breastfeeding.

How to Monitor Your Weight

You can do your own checkups on your weight gain during pregnancy. (Your prenatal health-care-giver will also do so during your periodic visits.)

1. Weigh yourself at the same time each week. Pick a time before a meal; before breakfast is popular.
2. After each weighing, write down the date and your weight (to the nearest half-pound or quarter-pound, if practical).
3. Compare your weight gain with the table here, "Rate of Weight Gain during Pregnancy," to tell if you are within the typical ranges.

Ask your care-giver about your weight if:

- you gain *more* than 2 pounds in any one week (and especially if you also have marked swelling of your face, hands, and feet); or
- you gain *less* than 2 pounds in any one month after your third month and before your ninth month.

As the table shows, some variations from the typical are nothing to worry about. But do be ready to question your care-giver for either of the reasons above. Most likely, there won't be a problem even then, since weight-gain patterns vary widely. Your care-provider will relate your gain to the size of your uterus. It's wise, though, to discuss whether you might need to adjust the foods and fluids you are consuming.

Rate of Weight Gain during Pregnancy (not Multiple Birth)

Time	Typical Rate of Gain	Typical Gain in Pounds	Percent of Total Gain (Cumulative)
1st 3 months	Minimal	0–4 lb	0–10%
4th month	1 lb/week	3–6 lb	15–25%
5th & 6th months	1+ lb/week	9–15 lb	40–60%
7th & 8th months	1 lb/week	8–14 lb	98–100%
9th month	Minimal	0–1 lb	100%
TOTAL		20–40 lb	

Why You Need a Hefty Weight Gain

Why should you gain 20 to 40 pounds for a baby who will weigh only about 7 or 8 pounds at birth? It's because only one-fifth to one-third of your total weight gain in pregnancy consists of the baby itself. The rest goes to make up the baby's life support systems—and the more efficient they are, the healthier your baby is likely to be.

You can see why it's important to gain enough weight from another table, "Sources of Weight Gain in Pregnancy." It shows the comparative weights of those vital life support systems for your baby.

Don't Resist Gaining Weight

That same "Sources of Weight Gain" table shows in addition why you should be able to return to just about your prepregnant weight fairly soon after the baby arrives.

37

Sources of Weight Gain in Pregnancy

	Pounds	Approx. % of Total Gain
Fetus	7–8 lb	35%
Placenta	1–2 lb	5%
Amniotic fluid	1–3 lb	5%
Uterine increase	2–5 lb	10%
Blood and body fluid increase	4–8 lb	20%
Breast increase	1–3 lb	5%
Fat and nutrient deposits	4–10 lb	20%
TOTAL	20–39 lb	100%

With birth itself, you'll shed the first three elements listed—the baby, plus the placenta and the amniotic fluid. Weight increases in the next two elements—your uterus, and your blood and body fluid—will be given off in not too many more weeks.

Only the weight increase in your breasts and in fat and nutrient deposits will last longer, and they total only some 5 to 13 pounds. You can probably whittle these extra pounds off in another month or so by postnatal exercise and avoidance of some extra calories in your diet.

In consequence, you need not be reluctant to put on a natural and substantial amount of weight in pregnancy for fear that you might have trouble losing it after your baby arrives. However, try not to use pregnancy as an excuse to indulge yourself with favorite high caloric foods.

How to Estimate Your Weight Gain

You can judge roughly whether your weight gain should be at the high or low end of the scale by looking at the table headed "Acceptable Weights for Women over 25 at LMP" (last menstrual period).

The closer your case comes to the top left of the table, the more likely that your weight gain should run near the lower of the 20-to-40-pound range we've talked about. Similarly, the closer you come to the bottom right of the table, the more likely your weight gain should run near the 40-pound upper end of the range.

If your weight is at least a few pounds more or less than the table shows for women of your height and frame, you may be overweight or underweight. In either case, you should ask your prenatal health-care-giver for advice on your weight gain and nutrition during pregnancy.

Acceptable Weights for Women over 25 at LMP*

Height Without Shoes	Type of Frame		
	Small	Medium	Large
4'8" (56")	92–98	96–107	104–119
4'9" (57")	94–101	98–110	106–122
4'10" (58")	96–104	101–113	109–125
4'11" (59")	99–107	104–116	112–128
5'0" (60")	102–110	107–119	115–131
5'1" (61")	105–113	110–112	118–134
5'2" (62")	108–116	113–126	121–138
5'3" (63")	111–119	116–130	125–142
5'4" (64")	114–123	120–135	129–146
5'5" (65")	118–137	124–139	133–150
5'6" (66")	122–131	128–143	127–154
5'7" (67")	126–135	132–147	141–158
5'8" (68")	130–140	136–151	145–163
5'9" (69")	134–144	140–155	149–168
5'10" (70")	138–148	144–159	153–173
5'11" (71")	142–152	148–163	157–177
6'0" (72")	146–156	152–167	161–181
6'1" (73")	150–160	156–171	165–185

Underweight: prepregnant weight 10% or more below standard weight for height and age†
Overweight: prepregnant weight 20% or more above standard weight for height and age†
* For women younger than 25, subtract 1 pound for each year under 25
† Roy M. Pitkin, "Risks Related to Nutritional Problems in Pregnancy" in *Risks in the Practice of Modern Obstetrics*, 2nd ed., Silvio Aladjem, Ed. (St. Louis: C. V. Mosby Co., 1975), p. 168. Reprinted with permission.
Source: This chart is reproduced, with permission, from the statement by the Medical Advisory Board of the Maternity Center Association entitled "Demonstration Project in Out-of-Hospital Maternity Care: Conditions Precluding Management at Childbearing Center."

Why Weight Gain Can Be Crucial

It is important for you to gain enough weight mainly in order to reduce the chances of having a low-birth-weight (LBW) baby. LBW babies, defined as weighing less than 5½ pounds (2,500 grams) at birth, run high risks:

- LBW babies exhibit a high death rate in their first year, 17 to 30 times higher than the rate for normal-weight infants. LBW babies account for about two-thirds of all babies who die before one month of age; they are 5 times more likely to die in the next 11 months of their lives than are infants of normal birth weight.

39

- If they survive, LBW babies have 10 times the chance of being mentally retarded compared to other babies. In a recent federal study, 50 percent of the children who had been LBW babies had IQs of less than 70 (100 IQ is average normal). But only 5 percent of comparable children with normal birth weights had IQs below 70.

    LBW babies also have physical conditions that make them much less vigorous, active, and alert at birth, and later more susceptible to infections and infant disorders such as colic, diarrhea, and anemia. Such weakened resistance may not be overcome in later life.

Eat the Right Foods

To achieve a weight gain that includes all the nutrients you and your baby need, follow this simple, basic plan for what to eat (and to drink—liquids count, too!). The plan is outlined in the "What to Eat and Drink Every Day."

Every day you should be sure to include choices from each of the seven food groups in the lefthand column for your meals and snacks. The *minimum* amounts you should have every day—in numbers of servings of normal size—are given in the righthand column.

What to Eat and Drink Every Day[3]

Food Group	Minimum Per Day
1. Milk or milk products (yogurt, cheese)	4 glasses (1 qt) of whole or skim milk, or equivalent in milk products
2. High-protein foods: meat, fish, eggs, and high-protein plant foods	4 servings, of which 1 may be 2 eggs (soybeans, beans, nuts, seeds, etc., if vegetarian)
3. Vegetables and fruits (or vegetable and fruit juices	4 to 5 servings, including 1 or 2 vitamin-C foods, and 1 or 2 dark-green leafy vegetables
4. Grains (whole-grain breads and cereals, brown rice, cornmeal, spaghetti, noodles)	4 to 5 servings
5. Fats and oils (butter or margarine, vegetable oil, mayonnaise, peanut butter)	2 servings (of about 1 tablespoon each)
6. Water	4 glasses (1 qt) or more
7. Vitamin & mineral supplements	Folic acid (vitamin B_9), 400–800 micrograms; iron, 30–60 milligrams

Just a few of the actual foods you can select from each of these food groups are identified in the following chart, "Examples of Foods You Can Choose in the Main Food Groups." Those examples show

Examples of Foods You Can Choose in the Main Food Groups

1. Milk and Milk Products (4 Servings Daily)

1 glass milk (8 oz)	1 cup ice milk	½ cup evaporated milk
1 cup yogurt	⅓ cup cottage cheese	⅓ cup powdered milk
1¼ oz hard cheese	1 cup ice cream	

2. High-protein Foods (4 Servings Daily)

2 eggs	2 slices lean ham	3 oz salmon
1 lean hamburger	3 oz turkey	2 slices meatloaf
1 medium fish patty	2 slices calves' liver	8 oz soybean curd (tofu)
1½ cups cooked dry peas or beans	3 oz Cheddar, Swiss, or other natural hard cheese	1 medium fish steak

3. Vegetables (2 to 3 Servings Daily) and Vegetable Juices

1 sweet potato	1 cup broccoli	1 cup asparagus
1 cup lettuce	1 cup spinach	1 potato
1 cup Brussels sprouts	1 cup green beans	1 cup beets
¾ cup cooked carrots	1 cup squash	1 ear corn
1 cup eggplant	1 cup cabbage	½ cup lima beans

3. Fruits (2 to 3 Servings Daily) and Fruit Juices

1 orange	5 dates	1 bunch grapes
½ grapefruit	1 banana	2 tangerines
½ cup strawberries	1 apple	1 cup papaya juice
½ cantaloupe	1 pear	½ cup raisins
2 oz dried apricots	1 peach	2 plums

4. Grains (4 to 5 Servings Daily)

1 slice wheat bread	½ cup noodles	1 pancake
½ muffin	½ cup oatmeal	½ cup rice
1 corn tortilla	½ English muffin	4–8 wheat crackers
½ cup whole-grain cereal	1 waffle, fruit topping	3 cups popcorn
	2 rice cakes	½ cup grits

5. Fats and Oils (2 Tablespoons Daily)

butter	vegetable oil	peanut butter
margarine	mayonnaise	sour cream

how you can pick out many varieties of appetizing foods to foster good health throughout pregnancy.

Unless you're normally on a low-salt diet, feel free to salt your food to taste while pregnant (with iodized salt or sea salt). But do *not* eat excess salt and junk foods such as:

- candy,
- potato chips, cheese chips, other chips,
- carbonated beverages, including colas,
- packaged pastries with many synthetic ingredients,
- heavily sugared pastries,
- large amounts of heavily salted french-fried potatoes, and
- sugar-coated cereals with many synthetic ingredients.

These load you with excess nonnutritive calories. Many may also contain chemical additives and preservatives that might impair the health of your baby.

If you drink cola beverages, remember that it's wise to limit caffeine-containing fluids to a glass or a cup or two a day, or better, not to have any, especially in the first three months of pregnancy.

Take Iron and Vitamin B$_9$ Supplements

Most care-givers will want you to take supplementary doses of certain vitamins and iron. Raise the question with your care-giver if he or she hasn't so advised.

The selection of foods you should eat daily, as shown in the table, is designed to give you vitamins and minerals that meet authoritatively defined RDA (Recommended Daily Allowance) amounts for pregnancy. You're especially likely to meet your vitamin and mineral needs if you eat mainly foods that are fresh or frozen (rather than canned or packaged varieties with preservatives and extra sweeteners and salt).

However, for two important exceptions—iron and vitamin B$_9$ (also called folic acid)—eating the recommended foods may not supply your RDA needs. You are therefore advised to take supplements in tablet form in at least the minimum daily amounts identified: 400 micrograms of vitamin B$_9$ and 30–60 milligrams of iron. (The higher ranges reflect the optimum daily amounts for some individuals due to variations in their physical constitutions and customary diets.)

These nutrients are crucial because without them your system cannot produce enough blood and red blood cells to nourish you and your baby well. Without enough of them, you can develop severe weakness and anemia that might seriously compromise you and the fetus.

There are two things you should know about iron in supplementary tablet form:

1. Take iron tablets after meals to minimize any digestive irritation they may cause; also, take them with orange juice (or some other acidic fruit juice) rather than with milk, because your system absorbs them best if you take them with an acidic liquid.

2. You need not be concerned about two aspects of taking iron tablets: first, any excess iron you take is simply thrown off by your system with no ill effects: second, taking iron may give your bowel movements a dark, tarlike appearance, which is harmless and normal.

Checklist to Help You Eat Properly Every Day

As a practical aid in following these guidelines, use the "Daily Nutritional Planning Checklist." It's designed for you to copy and use each day in two ways: (1) Fill it out for the next day as a guide to planning meals and snacks. (2) Each day, check off the items you had filled in the day before. The Checklist appears on page 44.

To illustrate just how to use the checklist, we give an example of one day's list filled in with selections you might make for that day.

Shopping for Foods

When shopping for foods of the main groups, follow these guidelines:

Group 1—Milk and Milk Products

Milk of any type will prove wholesome for you.

Flavor plain yogurt with fresh fruits, rather than buying preflavored types, which have excess calories in the form of sweeteners.

Choose natural hard cheeses—like Cheddar, Swiss, Muenster, and mozzarella—instead of processed cheese in order to avoid chemical additives.

Try to stick to the higher-quality types of ice cream and ice milk made with natural ingredients in order to avoid chemical additives.

Other milk products that are soundly nutritious include cottage cheese and natural soft cheeses, such as ricotta, Roquefort, Camembert, Brie, and Liederkranz.

Pregnancy

DAILY NUTRITIONAL PLANNING CHECKLIST

Water: Glasses (8-oz) to have (4 min) _____; did have _____

Breakfast: 1 serving fruit _____
1 serving milk (product) _____
1 serving grain _____

Snack: 1 serving fruit _____
1 serving milk (product) _____

Lunch: 1 serving milk (product) _____
1 serving protein _____
1 serving vegetable _____
1 serving grain _____

Snack: 1 serving protein _____
1 serving fruit _____
1 serving grain _____

Dinner: 1 serving protein _____
1 serving vegetable _____
1 serving grain _____
1 serving milk (product) _____
1 serving fruit dessert
    or _____
1 serving milk (product) dessert _____

Snack: 1 serving protein _____
1 serving grain _____

Iron: 1 tablet _____; Vitamin B$_9$ (folic acid), 1 tablet _____

Fats and Oils (2 tbsp): _____

SAMPLE FILLED-IN DAILY NUTRITIONAL PLANNING CHECKLIST

Water: Glasses (8-oz) to have (4 min) ____4____ ; did have ____5____

Breakfast: 1 serving fruit ____1 cup orange juice____ X
1 serving milk (product) ____1 cup milk____ X
1 serving grain ____½ cup oatmeal____ X

Snack: 1 serving fruit ____1 sliced peach____ X
1 serving milk (product) ____1 cup plain yogurt____ X

Lunch: 1 serving milk (product) ____1 cup milk____ X
1 serving protein ____cold ham or turkey____ X
1 serving vegetable ____lettuce and tomatoes____ X
1 serving grain ____bread sticks____ X

Snack: 1 serving protein ____3 oz Cheddar cheese____ X
1 serving fruit ____medium sized bunch grapes____ X
1 serving grain ____6 crackers____ X

Dinner: 1 serving protein ____broiled chicken____ X
1 serving vegetable ____broccoli____ X
1 serving grain ____brown rice____ X
1 serving milk (product) ____(dessert)____ X
1 serving fruit dessert
   or ____ice milk____ X
1 serving milk (product) dessert

Snack: 1 serving protein ____4 Tbsp peanut butter____ X
1 serving grain ____1 slice whole-wheat bread____ X

Iron: 1 tablet ____X____ ; Vitamin B$_9$ (folic acid), 1 tablet
____X____

Fats and Oils **(2 tbsp):** ____4 Tbsp peanut butter____ X

45

Group 2—High-Protein Foods: Meat, Fish, Eggs

Among meats, choose with two guidelines in mind:

1. Select leaner, less fatty meats such as chicken, turkey, and veal instead of beef or pork; liver is especially valuable because of its high iron content and little fat. (Leaner meats give you higher proportions of needed protein.)

2. Avoid large quantities of packaged meats such as cold cuts and frankfurters, since they may contain relatively large proportions of fats, nonmeat fillers, and preservatives.

Fish provide ample protein for few calories, but avoid sushi (raw fish) because of possible bacterial contamination.

Eggs serve as an excellent protein source.

Group 2—High-Protein Plant Foods

Much of the protein needed in pregnancy can be provided by plant foods, particularly such legumes as soybeans (which you can buy in health food stores raw, roasted, sprouted, or as soy flour or soy flakes), lentils, split peas, black-eye peas, kidney beans, peanuts, lima beans, navy beans, red beans, black beans, chick-peas (garbanzo beans), pinto beans, and tofu (soybean curd).

Combining most legumes with whole-grain foods (such as wheat or brown rice) or with milk products, provides you with much more protein than you would get from the legumes alone. Soybean foods, however, provide high-quality, high-quantity, and complete proteins all by themselves.

Nuts and seeds also supply substantial amounts of protein and some needed minerals (such as magnesium). Among just a few that are appetizing to eat separately or as toppings are alfalfa and alfalfa sprouts; sunflower seeds, pumpkin or squash seeds, sesame seeds; coconuts; and familiar nuts of all kinds—almonds, brazil nuts, filberts, pecans, pistachios, walnuts.

Some grains and vegetables give you moderate amounts of protein—for example, brown rice, whole-grain wheat bread, corn, and peas.

Group 3—Vegetables

Choose fresh vegetables over frozen or canned for their higher vitamin and mineral content. Eat vegetables raw or lightly cooked (steamed or boiled briefly). Long cooking reduces some nutrients by substantial amounts.

Green leafy vegetables are especially rich in vitamins and minerals; they're also convenient because most can be eaten raw, in salads. They include lettuce (dark-green varieties have more vitamins than the light-green iceberg type), spinach, chicory, escarole, Swiss chard, watercress, and cabbage.

Sweet potatoes, yams, and winter squash are especially good sources of iron and vitamin A.

Baked potatoes with the skins left on provide good nutrition (some vitamin C and iron), especially when served with a melted cheese topping for added protein.

Other unusually nutritious vegetables include asparagus, beets, broccoli, brussels sprouts, carrots (high in vitamin A), cauliflower, kale, green beans, greens (collard, dandelion, mustard, turnip), parsnips, peas, spinach, and tomatoes.

Vegetable juices can help meet your vegetable needs in a tasty and convenient way. (They're especially flavorful and nutritious when made from raw vegetables in your blender or juicer.)

Group 3—Fruits

Fruits and fruit juices provide good sources of quick energy (from natural sugars), vitamins, and iron.

Use fresh fruits and fresh (or frozen) fruit juices whenever possible, to avoid the extra sugar and chemicals often added to canned varieties.

Dried fruits like prunes, raisins, and apricots are good iron sources (and can help relieve mild constipation).

Substitute fresh fruits for pastry, candy, and junk foods.

Emphasize high-vitamin-C fruits, such as citrus fruits, mangoes, melons, pineapple, strawberries, and bananas.

Fruits high in vitamin A are also essential. They include apricots (dried), cantaloupe and watermelon, mangoes, nectarines, papayas, peaches, and prunes.

Group 4—Grains

Whenever possible, choose whole-grain items without chemical preservatives. "Cracked"-grain varieties are the next preference after whole-grain.

Examine ingredients lists on product labels to make sure that "whole grain" or "cracked grain" content is listed if that's what you're buying; don't be misled by vague promotional terms on the package, such as "natural" or "wheat."

Select enriched grain foods over nonenriched breads, cereals, and pasta. (Also, examine the ingredients list to choose on the basis of how much and what enrichment.)

Among nutritious grain foods to buy are whole-grain breads and rolls (100 percent whole wheat, rye); whole-grain flours (for pancakes, waffles, baking; buckwheat flour is whole-grain); wheat germ (for adding to cereals, beverages, stews and soups, and baked foods); and whole-grain cereals (hot or cold, such as oatmeal, 100 percent wheat porridge or flakes, or bran flakes or cereal biscuits).

Other good choices include brown rice; spaghetti, noodles, and other pasta made with whole-grain flour (or enriched unbleached white flour); and couscous (a Middle Eastern grain staple, fast-cooking and increasingly found in supermarkets).

Corn muffins, cornbread, and corn grits (or cornmeal mush) made from 100 percent cornmeal can provide you with much the same nutrients as whole-grain foods. Hominy grits (made from hulled corn) are not as nutritious as the whole-kernel corn cereals.

Group 5—Fats and Oils

Small amounts of fats and oils suffice (an aggregate of about 2 tablespoonfuls a day). Whenever possible, avoid chemical additives and preservatives.

Among especially nutritious fats and oils are butter; cream; sour cream; vegetable oil for cooking and salads (olive oil or 100 percent corn, peanut, safflower, or soybean oil without additives is preferable), kept refrigerated; peanut butter (natural or 100 percent peanut content); and mayonnaise.

Group 6—Water

You should drink at least 4 tall (8-ounce) glassfuls of water every day. Drink on up to even 6 or 8 a day for still greater benefits (in addition to the milk and juices you drink).

In many locales, however, tap water contains high levels of chemical pollutants that you would be wise to avoid (pollutants such as industrial wastes, fertilizer runoff, or, in very old buildings in some communities, lead from lead pipes). Home filtration units can be added to your water supply fairly simply and inexpensively, and prove effective. Bottled spring water is wholesome but more expensive. Distilled water may contain undesirable amounts of pollutants.

Recipes to Help You Eat Well Every Day

Certain dishes are particularly helpful or attractive during pregnancy. We offer several such recipes here as a further help in eating the right foods.

For Tasty Snacks—Quick and Refreshing

It's handy to be able to make something fast for snacks or for extra, light meals—and something that's really nourishing and delicious as well. Here are two suggestions.

Creamy Peanut-Date Pickup

¼ cup	boiling water
½ cup	natural peanut butter
1 cake	tofu (preferably soft)
½ cup	shelled peanuts
2 tablespoons	chopped dates
2 or 3	celery stalks (or whole-grain bread slices)

Add the boiling water to the peanut butter to form a creamy paste. Then add the tofu, mixing thoroughly. Add the peanuts and dates. Mix well, and spread on celery sticks (or on the bread, plain or toasted).

This is a quick, good energy source, high in protein and carbohydrates. ∎

Fruit-Yogurt Pickup

1 cup	plain yogurt
1 handful	seedless grapes
¼ cup	raisins
½ cup	chopped fresh peaches (or other fresh fruit)
⅛ cup	sunflower seeds
⅛ cup	unsalted nuts, chopped
¼ teaspoon	orange, lemon, or vanilla extract

Mix all the ingredients. ∎

A Quick, Satisfying Meal You Can Drink

Liquid meals can relieve both time pressures and digestive distress. Easily digested and light, they can help keep away those bloated, gassy, and constipated feelings that can come after eating too much that's hard to digest.

You can also make them as needed in very little time, or even ahead of time so that they're ready instantly when you need a meal.

You can make them up creatively from ingredients on hand: milk, plain yogurt, dried or fresh fruits, brewer's yeast (high in protein, iron, B vitamins), wheat germ, bran, honey, nuts, vanilla extract, and eggs (added raw in milk beverages).

Here's a recipe for one example of a tasty liquid meal.

Healthful Milkshake Meal

1 cup	milk
¼ cup	plain yogurt
2 tablespoons	wheat germ
½ tablespoon	chopped raisins
½ tablespoon	chopped walnuts
½	banana
to taste	honey or vanilla extract

Blend all ingredients until smooth. If you want, add a raw egg for still more protein. ∎

Breakfast Muffins to Beat Morning Sickness

One good way to head off or minimize morning sickness is to eat a highly nutritious, easily digested breakfast. You can center just such a breakfast around these muffins (rounding them out nutritionally with a large glass of fruit juice and a high-protein food like eggs or cottage cheese).

Apple-Walnut Breakfast Muffins

1 cup	whole-wheat pastry flour
¾ cup	bran
½ cup	raisins
¼ cup	chopped walnuts
½	large apple, chopped
⅛ teaspoon	salt
¾ teaspoon	baking soda
1 tablespoon	pure maple syrup (or barley malt)
⅛ cup	molasses

1 cup	plain yogurt (or buttermilk)
1	egg
1 tablespoon	cold-pressed oil

First mix the dry ingredients together. Then, separately, mix the liquid ingredients. Combine the two, stirring lightly. Pour into 12 greased muffin tins. Bake in a 350° oven for 20 to 30 minutes. ∎

Ideal Dish for a Light Dinner Meal

If you eat a light, easily digested dinner, deep, restful sleep through the night may come more naturally. This dish has excellent flavor, and any leftovers make a good snack.

Guacamole with Pita or Toast

2	avocados, pitted and mashed
2	cloves of garlic, pressed
1 tablespoon	minced green bell peppers
1 tablespoon	finely chopped onion (or scallions)
¼ teaspoon	cayenne pepper
2 tablespoons	fresh lemon juice

Mix ingredients well. Spoon into a piece of pita bread (or spread on toast). Garnish with toppings like shredded spinach or lettuce, sliced tomatoes, or alfalfa sprouts. ∎

For a Substantial Midday Dinner

More substantial, heavier meals on those demanding days when you need them might best be eaten as midday dinners. By eating substantially at noon and more lightly in the evening, you may be less likely to have a restless night while your system works away at digestion.

This recipe supplies you with a high-protein meal that's delicious as well.

Ratatouille Plus

1 cup	diced chicken meat (optional)
⅛ cup	olive oil
½	red bell pepper, sliced
½	green bell pepper, sliced
2	small zucchini, thinly sliced

1 cup	chopped string beans (or snow peas)
1 bunch	scallions, chopped
⅛ teaspoon	basil
⅛ teaspoon	oregano
2 cloves	garlic, pressed
2 cups	tomato sauce
2	baked potatoes, kept warm
1 cup	shredded Cheddar cheese

Sauté the diced chicken in the olive oil in a large skillet until lightly browned. Add the vegetables (but not the potatoes), spices, and tomato sauce and cook in an open pan over medium heat, 15 to 20 minutes or until tender, stirring occasionally. Cut the baked potatoes in half and mash their centers lightly. Pour the ratatouille over them, and sprinkle with the shredded cheese. Heat in a 300° oven until the cheese has melted. ■

Recommended Daily Allowances in Pregnancy

You can count on getting all the nutrients you need by eating as we've outlined here, if you're having a normal, low-risk pregnancy.

The nutrients needed in pregnancy are summed up more scientifically in the table on page 53 which presents the current RDAs as defined by the U.S. government.[4] Use the official RDAs as your guide if you're versed in nutrition. The values are designated for average persons and circumstances, and you might want to adjust them for your own system and activities. Adjustments like these can also be indicated by appetite and energy level.

Recommended Daily Allowances for Young Adult Nonpregnant, Pregnant, and Lactating Women

Nutrient and Units	Nonpregnant	Pregnant	Lactating
Protein (g)	44	+30	+20
Vitamin A (mg RE)	800	+200	+400
Vitamin D (mcg)	5	+5	+5
Vitamin E (mg and TE)	8	+2	+3
Vitamin C (mg)	60	+20	+40
Thiamin (mg)	1.0	+0.4	+0.5
Riboflavin (mg)	1.2	+0.3	+0.5
Niacin (mg)	13	+2	+5
Vitamin B_6 (mg)	2	+0.6	+0.5
Folacin (mcg)[b]	400	+400	+100
Vitamin B_{12} (mcg)	3.0	+1.0	+1.0
Calcium (mg)	800	+400	+400
Phosphorus (mg)	800	+400	+400
Magnesium (mg)	300	+150	+150
Iron (mg)	18	+30–60[a]	+30–60[a]
Zinc (mg)	15	+5	+10
Iodine (mcg)	150	+25	+50

[a] This intake cannot be met by the iron content of habitual American diets; the use of a supplement is recommended.

[b] Folacin has nutritional properties and chemical structure similar to folic acid.

Reprinted from "Recommended Dietary Allowances, Ninth Edition," 1980, with permission of the National Academy Press, Washington, D.C.

5

Avoiding Hazards and Coping with Common Complaints

Once the early developments of pregnancy are under way, you should make a number of decisions essential for the health and safety of your baby. You will also want to know how you can prevent or relieve the discomforts generally referred to as the "common complaints" of pregnancy.

Major Precautions to Take

Beginning in the early stages of pregnancy, it is very important for expectant parents to take certain precautions. These are precautions against harm to your unborn baby by injury (either from harmful substances or from physical actions) and by infection. Many women wonder whether activities in which they normally engage will be harmful or can be continued. Let's look first at commonly used substances that are of doubtful help or outright harm.

Alcohol

Babies born to mothers who drink heavily—women who typically drink more than four or five glasses of beer, wine, or mixed drinks a day—very often have serious abnormalities including mental retardation and physical deformities. Even though one occasional drink should do no harm, the safest course is to drink no alcohol whatever, especially during the first three months of pregnancy.

Smoking

Pregnant women who smoke tobacco endanger their unborn babies
in a variety of ways. Smoking increases the likelihood of low birth-
weight, with its accompanying higher health risks. Miscarriage, stillbirth, and hemorrhaging might also occur in extreme cases. The risks
are reduced by smoking substantially less. For the least risk, do not
smoke at all, and even avoid smoke-filled rooms (commonly referred
to as passive smoking). This may mean that your mate should cut
down sharply or smoke only out of your presence.

Caffeine

Caffeine in coffee, tea, hot chocolate or cocoa, and cola-type carbonated
beverages appears to present some risk of harm to unborn babies
when taken in large quantities—on the order of eight or more cups
of coffee a day. Mothers with high caffeine intake tend to have a
higher than normal incidence of difficulties like premature birth and
stillbirth. As a result, it's often advised to limit caffeine intake to as
little as a cup or glass or two of caffeinated beverages a day (or to
cut it out altogether, especially in the first trimester).

Drugs to Treat Mental Illness

When you are pregnant or trying to get pregnant, do not take tranquilizers, antidepressants, or any other drugs used to treat neurosis or
mental illness. Studies have shown that these drugs can result in
much higher chances of harm to your unborn baby. If you take any
drugs for mental or emotional therapy in pregnancy, do so only with
professional medical supervision and by prescription.

So Called "Recreational" or Other Drugs

During pregnancy be sure to take no do-it-yourself mood-changing
drugs whatever, such as marijuana, cocaine, heroin, LSD, angel dust,
speed (amphetamines), downers (barbiturates); also do not sniff glue
or amyl nitrite. In addition, for at least a month even before trying
to get pregnant, both you and your partner should stop taking any
such drugs.

Chances of harm to the unborn baby vary from one drug to another,
but studies often show alarming results. For your continued health,
it would be best to stay away from them completely—before, during,
and after pregnancy.

Medicines of All Kinds

Medicinal drugs of all varieties—whether over the counter, like aspirin, or prescribed, as in the case of antibiotics—can also have mild to very serious harmful effects on unborn babies. The accepted position today is that no medicinal drug of any kind that is taken by a pregnant woman can be assumed to be completely safe for her developing fetus. Accordingly, a pregnant woman should resort to medicinal drugs only when essential, and then only under professional supervision.

X-Rays and Anesthetics

X-rays can be extremely harmful to a woman's egg cells, as well as to a newly developing embryo or fetus. Authorities therefore urge that x-rays of the lower abdominal area of any woman of childbearing age—from puberty through menopause—be avoided unless absolutely necessary. The area should be screened if other parts of the body are x-rayed. It is strongly recommended that a woman who is pregnant or trying to become pregnant should not have any x-rays taken whatever, unless absolutely essential. If essential, the pregnancy must be well shielded. She should also be sure to avoid exposure to x-rays or radiation through other diagnostic techniques that use x-rays, such as fluoroscopy or CAT scans.

Similarly, a woman who is pregnant or possibly pregnant should avoid if at all possible any use of general anesthetics for surgery or dental work. Such anesthetics can act far more powerfully on the unborn baby than on the expectant mother. Even local anesthetics for dental work should be used with care, because they sometimes contain epinephrine, which constricts the blood vessels. Should surgery be necessary (women do get appendicitis and other ailments in pregnancy), regional or local anesthetics would be better.

Environmental Hazards in and out of the Home

Most kinds of work that expectant mothers have been doing in the workplace or at home can be continued almost up to the start of labor without danger to the unborn baby. In some jobs, however, the pregnant woman may find that her need for less strain and exertion, or her physical awkwardness, leads her to suspend working for a number of weeks before the due date.

By all means *ignore* the "old wives' tale" concerning physical activity that warns pregnant women against stretching their arms up higher than their shoulders. Behind this tale is an absolutely mistaken notion that such reaching pulls the umbilical cord tight around the neck of the fetus. You can see from examining Figure 7.3 that no such tightening could possibly happen.

On the other hand, certain jobs or work settings can pose hazards for unborn babies and should be given up as soon as pregnancy is recognized. If there are possibly hazardous metals or chemicals in your workplace (such as lead or lead dust), get professional advice on whether that situation is safe for you.

Work settings likely to expose women to higher than normal risks of pregnancy complications or birth defects are listed below, together with a brief description of the possible hazard. They are listed in random order, for illustrative purposes.

Work settings hazardous for pregnant employees	Reason for hazard
Motor vehicle toll booth	Possible excess exposure to lead in auto exhaust fumes
Nuclear power plant (man as well as woman)	Radiation exposure levels can be high enough to damage egg or sperm cells (lead-lined underpants can help protect)
Dry-cleaning plant	Possible excess exposure to benzene vapors, which can cause chromosome breaks
Facility manufacturing storage batteries, paint, or glass	Possible excess exposure to lead
Vinyl plastic manufacturing plant	Possible excess exposure to vinyl chloride, which leads to chromosome defects and higher death rates for fetuses, according to studies
Radio or TV transmitting equipment installation	Possible excess exposure to intense radio waves, which may impair the health of a fetus

Obtaining well-informed professional advice on possible hazards for expectant mothers in your workplace may prove difficult. The absence of research findings about possible harm from exposure to many thousands of common chemicals means that no one agency (not even the federal Occupational Safety and Health Administration) has completely reliable advice. However, the OSHA office in your area should be able to give you information and referrals that are of at least some help. Probably your best source of information about possible hazards would be a professional providing health care through pregnancy and birth who also has long experience in your locale.

Hazardous Chemicals

One widespread product to be cautious about during pregnancy is a disinfectant soap used in many hospitals, hexachlorophene. It is most widely known by the trade name "pHisoHex." Because of its apparent adverse effects on newborns, it is now marketed only for professional medical use, and hospitals no longer use it around infants or expectant mothers.

Hair dye is another kind of chemical that is possibly hazardous in pregnancy. Some studies indicate that certain compounds in permanent hair dyes cause a higher than normal incidence of damage to chromosomes in humans. Such chromosome damage can lead to higher risk of birth defects in fetuses, and has been found among women who dye their hair. The harmful chemicals are absorbed through the skin of the scalp. The best choice would be not to use hair dye of the permanent type during pregnancy, or even throughout your child-bearing years.

As further examples, common chemicals (or types of chemicals) to avoid are identified in the following list.

Mercury	Met more often as a medical or industrial compound (calomel, mercurous chloride) than in pure form; overexposure leads to cerebral palsy, blindness, and brain damage in newborns.
Cadmium	A component in tobacco smoke, it also occurs in wastes from electroplating plants and is given off into the air by wearing or burning tires; seems to retard growth and increase deformities in fetuses.
Carbon monoxide	Extended exposure to high concentrations met in auto traffic jams tend to lower birth-weights and increase infant mortality rates.
Ozone	An oxygen variant occurring in high concentrations in smog, and also in airliners at high altitudes; flight stewardesses have blamed this for their occupationally high incidence of miscarriages and birth defects.

Pesticides . . . . Of 1,500 active ingredients in pesticides registered with the Environmental Protection Agency, the EPA says that 25 percent promote chromosome damage and cancer; only very few (such as DDT and chlordane) have had their use limited by the EPA, but partial evidence strongly suggests that excess exposure to any one of a great many pesticides may permanently harm fetuses.

Uranium wastes . . . . Uranium mining wastes were long used in Colorado to build roads and house foundations, while similarly radioactive slag was made into cinder blocks used to build homes in many other states. Rains draining through uranium mining wastes have made the drinking water in parts of Colorado, New Mexico, Utah, and other states abnormally radioactive. Such heightened radiation increases the incidence of birth defects and miscarriages.

Anesthetic gases . . . . Anesthetists, nurses, aides, and surgeons working in hospital operating rooms have abnormally high rates of sterility, miscarriage, and birth deformities; excess exposure to anesthetic gases seems to be the cause. A study by the American Society of Anesthesiologists urged as a result that pregnant women be kept out of operating rooms.

Solvents (analine, toluene, turpentine) . . . These solvents, used in industry as well as in arts and crafts, are viewed as hazardous during pregnancy in the case of long exposure to constant high concentrations.

PCBs . . . . PCBs (polychlorinated biphenyls) were once widely used for electrical insulation in transformers and other devices as well as for other purposes in many other common products. So dangerous are PCBs as carcinogens that the EPA banned their production in the U.S. in 1979. However, PCB wastes remain where dumped on river bottoms, and PCB-containing products will continue to be scrapped and to release PCBs into water and food supplies for many years ahead. Some authorities advise pregnant women to reduce their chances of ingesting PCBs by not eating freshwater fish, nor bottom-feeding fish like flounder and sole. Babies whose mothers accidentally ate high concentrations of PCBs in pregnancy have had high rates of eye and tooth defects and other abnormalities.

Dioxin derivatives . . . . Herbicides (which often have long scientific names revealing the component dioxin—2,3,7,8-tetrachlorodibenzo-p-dioxin, for instance) tend to be highly toxic in large quantities, and even in amounts safe for adults seem to cause abnormally high incidence of miscarriage. This was indicated in a 1979 EPA study of spontaneous abortions occurring after dioxin spraying of Oregon forests to increase timber production.

Infection

Unborn babies generally run little risk of harm from infectious diseases that their expectant mothers have caught. Exceptions especially important for you to know about are noted here.

German measles: German measles, or rubella, is usually a mild childhood disease in which a youngster mainly runs a low fever and develops a rash. However, if a woman in about the first five months of pregnancy catches it for the first time, the fetus has a very high probability of developing serious birth defects.

As a result, prenatal care-providers will usually screen your blood for antibodies to the disease at your first visit. But even if you're only thinking of having a child, it's wise to determine whether you've had rubella and have thereby gained complete immunity. Many adults had it as children. If you didn't, you should be vaccinated and then make certain not to become pregnant for at least three months, until immunity does develop.

In a pregnancy, if blood test results are positive, and you haven't had rubella since conceiving, everything's probably fine. If negative (demonstrating you have not had rubella), you should avoid contact with children of about age 12 or younger (who might be likely to have rubella). And should you be exposed to it, seek professional medical help, which might include the prescribing of gamma globulin in an attempt to protect you from developing the disease.

Toxoplasmosis: Serious birth defects or difficulties can also stem from the parasitic disease toxoplasmosis. Simple precautions can protect against it. Raw or almost raw meats are one source of the parasites, and should not be eaten. The parasites of toxoplasmosis can also exist in cat litter or droppings, which should be handled not at all or only with extreme caution. Blood tests can determine whether or not you have been exposed.

High fevers: A case of the flu or a sore throat usually would not directly harm your unborn baby. But if any illness brings on a fever, try to keep your temperature from rising higher than 102° (by means of cool baths and rest rather than medication, if possible), and check immediately with your care-provider. There are some indications in research studies that high fevers in the early weeks of pregnancy can have harmful effects on the fetus.

Sexually transmitted diseases: In most states, laws require that pregnant women be given a blood test for syphilis—and be given immediate treatment if it is found, so that the baby will be protected.

If an expectant mother has contracted gonorrhea, she of course should be treated immediately. Additional measures to protect the baby can be taken at the time of birth (gonorrhea is not transmitted through the placenta). The risk of the infant contracting gonorrhea in its eyes as it passes through the birth canal can be eliminated by administering eye drops within the first few hours of birth. Use of such antibiotic or silver nitrate eye medications is required by law for all babies in many states.

If the mother is found to have another major venereal disease, genital herpes (herpes simplex virus II), measures to protect the baby can also be taken at birth. Active herpes lesions in the birth canal when labor starts will necessitate delivery by cesarean section in order to prevent serious infection at birth.

One pioneering type of procedure to screen for active herpes II lesions in the birth canal has so far proven very effective. If the expectant mother has had lesions in the past, weekly herpes cultures are done starting in the fifth week before the expected delivery date. (Tests involve quickly and painlessly taking specimens at multiple birth-canal sites in a medical examining room and analyzing the specimens immediately in an adjacent lab with live tissue cultures.)

Results have proven far more reliable than with other types of screening methods, and are more rapidly available—on the day after testing. Only 14 percent of the women at risk with whom it has been used have proven to have had active herpes when labor started, and have required cesarean section. Remarkably, the other 86 percent could proceed safely with normal vaginal deliveries, insofar as herpes was concerned. The procedure is called "sequential monitoring for genital herpes simplex."[1] Should you require screening, inquire at larger hospitals or medical centers in your area. This type of monitoring is expensive.

AIDS: In the early 1980s concern developed, especially in New York and a few other cities, over possible pregnancy hazards raised by the outbreak of an epidemic of AIDS (acquired immunity deficiency syndrome). It is a condition in which the affected individual suffers from a breakdown in the body's immune system, which protects against infections. AIDS appears to have an extraordinarily high fatality rate with death caused by infections against which the victims' systems have lost their defenses. There is a great deal yet to be learned about the condition and its impact on childbearing.

Only persons who are members (or sexual partners of members) of groups identified as having an increased risk of getting AIDS need to be concerned at this time, according to public health officials. These groups include sexually active homosexual or bisexual men, persons using intravenous street drugs, and hemophiliacs receiving periodic blood transfusions.

Those who think they may be at increased risk of getting AIDS should seek advice from public health departments experienced in dealing with the disease, and from their care-provider. New information is being reported regularly.

Physical Activities

Sexual relations: If desired, sexual intercourse can usually be continued without risk through the last weeks and days of pregnancy. However, certain precautions should be observed as pregnancy progresses. As mentioned earlier, it may be desirable to alter positions in order to avoid placing weight directly on the woman's abdomen, especially in the last months of pregnancy. Side positions, including vaginal entry from a position at the woman's back, represent examples of such alternatives.

Avoid intercourse if vaginal spotting of blood occurs and inform your care-giver. The discharge of blood-tinged mucus from the vagina just a few weeks or less before the due date need not call for special precautions. (This is the "show," consisting of mucus that had sealed the cervix along with some blood from small capillaries that ruptured as the cervix began to dilate and efface—that is, open and thin. The discharge often occurs shortly before labor begins.)

If you have had trouble with premature labor in a prior pregnancy, it would probably be wise for you to seek professional advice on special precautions regarding intercourse.

Sports and athletics: Expectant mothers who are in good health and who have been active in recreational sports can usually continue in their athletic pursuits. Be sensible. It's wise not to push too hard or to get overtired. It's also wise not to overstrain parts of the body already under extra loads, like the back (particularly the lower back), the abdominal wall, the legs, knees, ankles, and feet, and the heart and circulatory system.

Hiking (without heavy backpacks and avoiding treacherous trails) and swimming are especially good sports for pregnant women. Jogging can usually be continued if you engaged in it prior to pregnancy, but needs to be done with care for the back and legs and without becoming badly winded or exhausted. Tennis or golf might be continued, again with care to avoid wrenching the back or getting exhausted. With skiing or water-skiing, it's probably most sensible to say no for the time being and thus run no risk of a fall—which might be more injurious to you than to your unborn baby.

Swimming or taking a tub bath does not expose the unborn baby to any threat of infection from water entering the uterus through the vagina. With baths, though, take special care not to use extremely hot water and of course not to slip and fall. Stay out of saunas and hot tubs while pregnant. Studies have shown that soaking in a hot tub for ten or fifteen minutes can raise a woman's internal temperature to levels believed to be hazardous to the central nervous system of a fetus.

Well modulated conditioning exercises are not only generally allowed but are strongly recommended. Certain exercises are extremely valuable during pregnancy (see Chapter 10). However, do not do sit-ups or leg-raises, both of which are exercises you would carry out while lying on your back. Either exercise might cause a separation in your abdominal wall muscle, which is already heavily stressed during pregnancy.

Women with health conditions such as heart disease, high blood pressure, diabetes, or kidney disease should obtain professional medical advice on sports activity and exercise during pregnancy. It may be advisable for them to restrict or suspend athletic pursuits, depending on specific factors in their condition.

Common Complaints—and How to Relieve Them

Quite normal and minor physical discomforts or difficulties may develop in early pregnancy. They result very naturally from the physical changes in the pregnant woman, which begin with conception and the initial growth of the baby. There are a number of remedies for these discomforts, traditionally termed "common complaints."

The Digestive and Genito-Urinary Systems

Nausea, or "morning sickness": Nausea or a queasy feeling in your stomach (possibly with vomiting) starting in the early weeks of pregnancy is fairly common. Although called morning sickness, it is felt by quite a few women not only in the morning but early in the evening or at other times of the day. A number of women—perhaps as many as half or more—do not get it at all, or get it only slightly. The nausea usually lessens and ends after about the third month of pregnancy. Its causes have not yet been determined, but it is thought to result in part from changes in body chemistry.

You may want to use one or more of these remedies, which usually bring substantial relief:

- Eat a few dry crackers (or another light, bland food like dry toast or unbuttered popcorn) twenty to thirty minutes before you get up in the morning.
- Move slowly and calmly—without rush or pressure—when you do get up; rise a quarter-hour or more earlier than usual to allow for this.
- Just before bedtime (or when getting up during the night), eat a palatable high-protein snack like cheese with some fruit or juice, or a glass of milk with toast.
- Avoid greasy, fried, or fatty foods, especially for breakfast. At breakfast, try to have acidic juices or fruits at the end of the meal. Some pregnant women find it helpful to avoid very spicy or sweet foods.
- Drinking nonacidic juices or carbonated beverages may relieve mild nausea.
- Keep some food and liquid in your stomach at all times by having four to six smaller meals, or by eating nutritious snacks between meals.

If simple remedies like these fail to bring relief from nausea or vomiting, seek professional advice. However, try to avoid taking any antinausea drugs; as with any drugs, they may harm the unborn baby. Some mothers have found that these drugs have little or no effect in easing the distress of nausea during pregnancy.

Constipation: A pregnant woman may become constipated at times, due at least partly to the new pressures on her abdominal organs. (It may also be caused by her own increased secretion of "relaxin," a substance causing smooth muscle, like that in the uterus and the bowel, to relax.)

Try eating more whole-grain cereals and breads, dried fruits, fresh fruits, and raw vegetables. Abundant water and other liquids are important, too. Also try more exercise, such as a daily walk, and try holding to a regular time of the day to attempt elimination (and don't be worried if you can't have a bowel movement on some days, so long as the movements you do have are not hardened and therefore don't require you to strain).

Heartburn: In the later months of pregnancy you may more often experience heartburn, with its feeling of burning and acidity deep down in your throat. It occurs because your stomach empties more slowly during pregnancy, and food and digestive juices can back up into the esophagus.

To relieve heartburn there are several possible remedies. Again, try eating smaller and more frequent meals. Eat more slowly and chew thoroughly to promote good digestion. Substitute foods you can digest more easily for those that you find harder to digest, such as very spicy or very fatty foods. Be guided in your choices by your own reactions to them.

Hemorrhoids: Hemorrhoids are swollen and sore blood vessels around and within the anal opening. In pregnancy, they may develop partly because of increased pressure on these veins and on the lower abdomen and pelvis generally.

You might relieve or perhaps even prevent hemorrhoids by avoiding long stints of sitting or standing. They can be aggravated (or even caused) by straining heavily while trying to have a bowel movement. They can usually be relieved or prevented by eating the foods that promote easy bowel movements (whole-grain foods, fresh fruits and vegetables, bran cereal, and stewed prunes).

Other measures include drinking more liquids and doing pelvic-floor-muscle exercises (see Chapter 10). Another helpful exercise is to lie on your back, with knees bent and a pillow under your hips, and hold your anal muscles tight for several seconds at a time, relax, and repeat 10–15 times.

When you must sit for a long time, sit on a firm chair instead of a soft cushion, or sit on the floor in the cross-legged yoga position called the lotus. You can relieve any severe itching and swelling with warm baths, ice packs, or cold compresses soaked in witch hazel.

Urinary pressures and infections: Early and again late in pregnancy, the uterus presses on the bladder and causes a need to urinate frequently. It is important to respond to this need and to empty the bladder as completely as possible on each occasion. Not emptying the bladder as need arises may contribute to infections of the bladder or the urinary tract (evidenced by burning or stinging sensations while urinating). This can lead to a serious kidney infection. To help prevent infection, drink large amounts of water and other liquids. If you develop an infection, seek treatment without delay, because it may intensify rapidly.

Excess saliva: This condition, properly called ptyalism, develops in a very small proportion of women during pregnancy. It is not harmful in any way but can be extremely annoying. Severe cases may require frequent use of tissues or cups to dispose of the excess saliva. The problem ends without any aftereffects when pregnancy is over.

The Muscular System and the Need for Sleep

Sleepiness: Your system's overall need for sleep can increase by as much as several hours a day in the first three months of pregnancy. Your body needs additional sleep because of the energy consumed by the rapidly growing fetus, the formation of the placenta, and the many other accommodations developing in your body. Getting added sleep is important to your health (and the baby's) and should not be viewed as laziness or neurotic behavior.

Get the extra sleep you need by going to bed earlier at night and by taking naps. If you're working, a nap at lunchtime or snacks of fruit or whole-grain crackers can provide quick energy. Make allowances for sometimes feeling impatient, irritable, or unable to concentrate due to fatigue.

Tiredness comes to an end for many women after the third month, and they go on to feel full of energy. If high levels of fatigue continue on into the fourth month, consider being checked for possible anemia.

A feeling akin to the tiredness experienced in early pregnancy is a shortness of breath felt by many women in the later months of pregnancy. It develops because the mother is literally breathing for two—her lungs are providing the oxygen for the unborn baby as well as herself. Moreover, the enlarged uterus is pressing up on the diaphragm and reducing the space in the rib cage in which the lungs can expand. Nature does compensate by permitting wider expansion of the rib cage—many women notice an increase in chest size as well as an enlargement of the breasts during pregnancy.

To cope with a sense of shortness of breath, move more slowly and breathe more deeply. It's also wise to take several deep breaths before getting out of bed in the morning. During prolonged sitting, raising the shoulders for several breaths from time to time can relieve the feeling.

Leg cramps: Increasing pressure placed on blood vessels to the legs by the enlarging uterus and fetus can lead to cramps in the leg, particularly in the calf. Cramps in the calf can be relieved by slowly stretching the calf muscle, in any of a number of ways.

For example, if you're standing, put the toes of the cramped leg on the edge of a securely placed chair seat and slowly move your heel downward to stretch the cramped calf muscle. Repeat several times until the cramp goes away. Or lean forward against a wall with your leg stretched behind, heel on the floor, so that the greatest possible stretch is put on the cramped muscle. Sometimes just walking around can "break" the cramp. If the cramp comes at night in bed, get close to the footboard or a wall and push with your feet flat against it. Pushing several times like this should relieve the cramp.

Your partner can also help relieve your leg cramps. Lie down with your legs straight, knees unbent. Your partner then gently bends your foot at the ankle so that the toes move upward, closer to your head, as illustrated in Figure 5.1. Repeating this a few times ought to end the cramp. The principle, always, is to stretch the cramped muscle. Massaging the cramp is not the answer.

You can help prevent cramps by lying down several times a day with your legs propped up higher than your head.

Backache: Backaches often result from poor posture. You should be able to prevent lower-back pain by holding yourself erect and letting your pelvic bones, rather than your back or your abdominal muscles, carry most of the weight of your growing uterus (see Figures 7.4 through 7.7 in Chapter 7).

One way of relieving backache is to sit on the floor or on a bed in a position like the lotus in yoga, but instead of crossing your legs, hold them with the soles of your feet touching (this is sometimes called

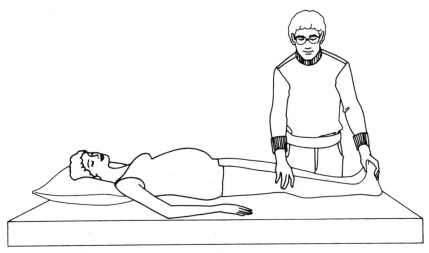

Figure 5.1. Stretch calf muscles to relieve leg cramps

"tailor-sitting"). The "pelvic rock" exercise (Figure 10.1) also gives relief (see Chapter 10), as does sleeping on your side with pillows between your knees (see Figures 7.9 and 7.10). The principle is to take the strain off muscles and ligaments, particularly the utero-sacral ligament (pictured in Figure 5.2), which connects the lower rear of the uterus to the backbone.

Abdominal muscle aches: Aches and twinges in abdominal muscles may be felt in the later months of pregnancy. They can be prevented or minimized by doing prenatal exercises, as described in Chapter 10, to give those muscles strength and tone. When they do occur, they result from the heavy load carried by the abdominal muscles and ligaments. Remedies include sitting or lying down briefly until they go away. Serious problems with an aching abdominal wall might justify use of an abdominal support or maternity girdle for relief of pressure.

Along with aches in the abdominal muscles, some women experience pain or aching in the vulva—more often on the right than the left side—sometimes giving the sensation that the vaginal outlet is opening. This is caused by the fact that, in most women, the uterus tends to be located not exactly on the midline but more on the right side. The vulvar ache is caused by tension on one of the round ligaments, which originate high up on each side of the uterus and terminate in the vulvar tissues, as shown in Figure 5.2.

You can relieve such aches with the same remedies you would use for aches in the abdominal muscles—by sitting or lying down until

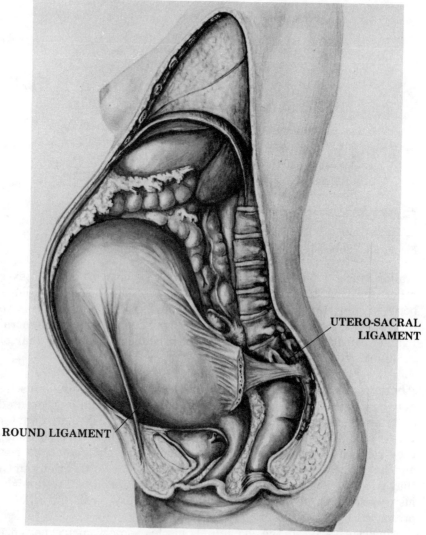

UTERO-SACRAL
LIGAMENT

ROUND LIGAMENT

Figure 5.2. The uterus in the ninth month of pregnancy

the ache stops, or by using a maternity girdle if it persists and hurts badly.

The Blood and Circulatory System

Anemia: An expectant mother who feels extremely tired at all times and gets exhausted after even modest physical effort may have anemia.

In this condition, a deficiency of iron leads to a lessening in the ability of the red blood cells to carry oxygen to the tissues (and consequent insufficient nourishment and energy for the body cells of both herself and the unborn baby). The normal increase in maternal blood volume can cause some anemia just by its diluting effect on blood contents.

You can usually prevent or correct anemia by including sufficient iron in your diet. A woman is generally thought to need about 2 to 3 times as much iron in her diet after she becomes pregnant. (Chapter 4 tells how you can get enough through iron-rich foods and iron-pill supplements.)

Be sure to watch out for anemia during pregnancy and to treat it promptly and effectively should it develop.

Vaginal bleeding and vaginal discharge: About 1 in every 4 or 5 women have some vaginal bleeding in the first trimester of pregnancy. You should tell the practitioner providing your prenatal care about any such bleeding. However, it probably doesn't indicate any serious trouble if the amount is minor and you have no pain along with it. As mentioned before, a bloody vaginal mucus discharge late in pregnancy, within a few weeks of your due date, often serves as a normal sign of approaching labor. *But any bleeding from the vagina should certainly be reported to your care-giver.*

Vaginal bleeding should not be confused with the vaginal discharge that often increases substantially with pregnancy. The discharge consists largely of clear and pale mucus, which is being produced by the cervix and the lining of the vagina in greater amounts than when you are not pregnant.

Varicose veins: Women may develop varicose veins in their legs during the later months of pregnancy as a result of the action of hormones on smooth muscle throughout the body, or because of pressures on blood vessels that return blood flow from the legs. These pressures can also bring on cramps in leg muscles, as mentioned earlier. Varicose veins may be relieved or prevented by reducing the pressures imposed by the weight of the unborn baby.

- Avoid standing or sitting for long periods of time without a break.
- When sitting, try to prop your feet up on a footstool as often as possible (or if you work at a desk, on a desk footrest or wastebasket), as shown in Figure 5.3.
- Get up and walk about frequently, if practical.
- Lie down often with your feet propped up higher than your head.

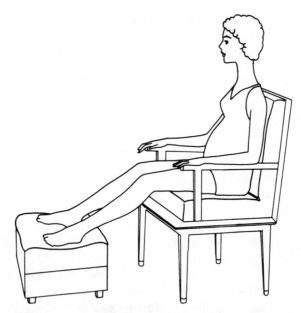

Figure 5.3. Sit with feet propped up to prevent varicose veins

This can relieve the blood congestion in your legs that produces or aggravates varicose veins. It may be helpful to lie down with your legs resting almost straight up against a wall for five to ten minutes or so before going to bed for the night. If propping helps, you might want to consider placing pillows or folded blankets between your mattress and the box spring to elevate the foot of the bed. (This is easier than trying to keep your legs on pillows during sleep.)

• Get regular exercise like walking or swimming. Doing so can improve blood circulation in the legs.

• Wear support hose if varicose veins are particularly severe in your case.

• Seek professional advice for still more countermeasures if needed.

You'll recall that hemorrhoids are essentially varicose veins occurring near the anal opening. They will tend to be relieved by the actions that ease varicose veins. Vulvar varicose veins can also occur and may be relieved by using a maternity support to reduce downward pressure.

Nosebleeds and other mucous-membrane problems: The increased blood volume that develops in pregnancy circulates actively in the mucous membranes and may sometimes result in nosebleeds, as well as congestion or stuffiness in the nose. It can also lead to swollen and puffy gums, and to redness and teariness of the eyes. Therefore nosebleeds and stuffiness can be a symptom of increased blood levels and activity in the mucous membranes rather than cold or allergy.

Avoid using nasal decongestants or antihistamines, which might adversely affect your baby.

The Skin and Skin Tissues

Stretch marks and other coloration changes: In many women, a few light-reddish lines or streaks, spaced at wide intervals on the stretched skin of the abdomen, appear in the later months of pregnancy. These are called stretch marks. They may also appear on the breasts, hips, or thighs. After the baby is born they become faint and turn a whitish or silvery color. Views differ on whether or not they can be prevented. Some authorities believe they may be minimized or perhaps prevented by periodic, gentle massaging of the skin with cocoa butter, oil, or lotion, and by taking vitamin E or applying it to the skin.

Among other possible changes in skin coloration is the development of slightly darkish patches on the face, called the mask of pregnancy, which occurs in a few expectant mothers and usually disappears after the baby is born. These patches may also appear on the neck or abdomen; they darken with suntan. In black women, they appear as paler skin patches. They are thought by some authorities to result from a folic acid deficiency. Discuss the adequacy of your folic acid intake with your care-provider if you have this condition.

A dark line extending from the navel down to the pubic area (called the *linea nigra*) may appear. In addition to the areola of the breast, the external genitalia may darken. All these colorations usually disappear when pregnancy ends.

Two other changes in skin coloration that occur in small numbers of women are delicate, reddened traceries of the tiny blood vessels called capillaries, and reddened palms of the hands. Both conditions bring no discomfort and have no harmful effects whatever, and both usually vanish entirely after pregnancy ends. The traceries, or vascular "spiders," consist of tiny reddish raised spots from which thread-marks run out a short distance like spokes of a wheel. These tend to appear on the arms, upper chest, neck and face. The condition of reddish palms is termed palmar erythema.

73

Swelling: It is quite normal and healthy in pregnancy to have a small or minimal amount of swelling in the skin tissues of the ankles, feet, wrists, hands, and sometimes the face, caused by retention of fluid. Increased fluid in the system peaks at about the seventh month, and the feeling of fullness which accompanies increased blood volume often declines thereafter.

Avoid tight-fitting cuffs, footwear, bracelets, or rings for comfort with the normal amounts of swelling. Use as much salt on your food as you ordinarily do, for cutting your salt intake may increase rather than decrease the swelling.

If such swelling should increase suddenly, become excessive, or cause unusual weight gain, ask those providing your prenatal care about it. Question any advice you may receive about taking a diuretic, or water-reducing medication, for such swelling (called edema). Diuretics were once widely prescribed for the condition during pregnancy. However, the U.S. Food and Drug Administration has issued a ruling that taking diuretics during pregnancy may be harmful because they reduce blood circulation to the placenta.

As indicated, any number of the so-called common complaints may occur during the childbearing process. While they are generally manageable, any unusual persistence should be called to the attention of your care-provider.

6

ᐩᐧᔕᐩᐧᔕ

Appropriate Use of Advanced Technologies

The tension between technologic and humanistic concerns in health care is obvious to all of us. We support the appropriate use of technology—but appropriate use is not always easy to determine, particularly in this day of increasing numbers of lawsuits. A defensive practice phenomenon has resulted. Diagnostic and even surgical procedures are recommended in the belief that they will lessen the likelihood of suits brought from malpractice. Therefore you need to collect as much information as you can from all sources and preferably in advance of being confronted with the need to make a decision.

In general, our belief is that technology should be used when it can provide necessary information or safety not available through more conventional means. For example, we do not have an electronic fetal monitor in the Childbearing Center. In our estimation, it has not been proven superior to a well-prepared human care-giver using a stethoscope, and its use does put undesirable constraints on the activities of the laboring woman.

There may be important advantages to the use of technologic methods if you really need them. On the other hand, these technologies might risk needless injury or infection for yourself or your unborn baby if used without sufficient justification, or if applied by care-givers not completely familiar with their proper use.

Much controversy has arisen over routine use of certain advanced technologies. In particular, many health-care professionals argue for the routine use of ultrasound scans, or sonograms, and of electronic fetal monitoring tests in late pregnancy for what might be considered high-risk pregnancies. Some of these professionals also recommend amniocentesis for routine or minor reasons, such as determining the sex of the fetus. Professionals with views like these tend to minimize the risk potential and to emphasize the possible advantages.

Other health-care professionals criticize the use of these technologies for routine or relatively unimportant reasons, such as convenience. They urge that these and any other technologic methods be employed in childbearing only after the expectant parents actively decide the question, based on full information from their care-givers. The parents' decision should be founded on the judgment that the specific advantages to be gained clearly outweigh the risks necessarily involved in the use of a particular technology.

Deciding on Ultrasound Scans

Your physician or other professional providing prenatal care might advise that you have an ultrasound scan, or sonogram, for reasons ranging from very important to quite casual ones.

An ultrasound scan provides images of structures inside the body like those obtained by x-ray machines. Compared to x-rays, though, ultrasound scans have two advantages: first, they do not employ x-rays (which have been shown to act as a cancer-inducing agent, or carcinogen, in large or long exposures); and second, they provide images of various kinds of soft tissues, including fetal tissues, as well as of skeletal tissues.

These scans are made by equipment that generates sound waves much higher in frequency than the range you can hear. A frequency of up to 2 million cycles a second is generated on some equipment (compared to about 15,000 cycles for the highest audible sound waves), and hence, the scans are called ultrasonic or ultrasound. They are not inexpensive; a test can cost over $100.

Specialists are able to use the images produced by the scans for a number of purposes. One, mentioned in an earlier chapter, is to estimate the due date for the baby's delivery (this can be done no earlier than around the eighth week of pregnancy). Other purposes include examining the fetus for its size and position and for possible birth defects, and determining the position of the placenta. Sonography is also necessary for the performance of amniocentesis.

Scans can be used for early detection of multiple fetuses. The opportunity to learn the sex of the fetus (which is possible only after fifteen weeks of gestation) serves as an incidental purpose for persons having a scan made for other, more important reasons. There's a fair likelihood that scans may be recommended almost as a matter of routine—perhaps as often as every few weeks—simply to assess the fetus's development.

Some practitioners giving prenatal care may recommend ultrasound scans for unnecessary purposes, such as allowing you to see your unborn baby kicking after the eighth week of pregnancy, or making breathing motions after the sixteenth week. There are other and better ways for you to become acquainted with your growing baby.

You should be cautious about scans for one major reason: Although no injury to the fetus or expectant mother appears to result from the technique in the first few months or years after the baby's birth, the technique has not been available long enough for anyone to know what its long-range effects may be. Some types of prenatal technology originally assumed to be safe have been dropped in recent decades. For example, early x-ray examination of the woman's pelvis for adequacy (size for delivery) is no longer done because of the effects on the growing baby.

If you decide that the reasons for having an ultrasound scan are extremely important, you will find that the procedure is not particularly inconvenient or uncomfortable. You will be required to go to a medical office and to drink a large amount of water to fill your bladder. In an examining or treatment room, an ultrasound specialist (also called a diagnostic medical sonographer) or your care-giver will have you lie down on an examining table and expose your abdomen. A small hand unit like a phone receiver or microphone is passed over the abdominal area, resulting in shadowy images on a TV-like screen. The images can also be recorded as photographs.

Shown in the images will be various parts of the fetus and your internal organs. You would probably not be able to recognize anything on your own. Ultrasound scan images resemble photographs only to a very slight extent, and require extensive professional background for correct interpretation.

Deciding on Amniocentesis

Amniocentesis is commonly used to determine whether the fetus has a serious genetic birth defect. Your prenatal care-giver might recommend use of the technique (and perhaps also advise you to consult a genetics counselor, and expert on dealing with possible hereditary birth defects) if one of the following circumstances applies to you:

- You have previously given birth to a child with a genetic birth defect that amniocentesis can diagnose (possibly including Down syndrome).
- Your family or ethnic group has a history indicating special susceptibility to genetic birth defects, such as Tay-Sachs disease.
- You have taken illegal drugs such as LSD or cocaine, have consumed excessive alcohol, have been x-rayed, or have been exposed to German measles (rubella) since becoming pregnant.

You may want to consider amniocentesis only if you are willing (or think you might be willing) to lose the baby. For one thing, the technique poses a slight risk (1 chance in 200 to 500) of infection, hemorrhage, or miscarriage. In addition, the usual purpose for having amniocentesis is to discover with more than 99 percent certainty whether or not the fetus has a serious hereditary birth defect. If you would not be willing to terminate your pregnancy whatever the findings, there would be no point in running the slight risks of amniocentesis.

On the other hand, findings from amniocentesis can bring great relief to an expectant couple when the test shows that their unborn baby does not have a birth defect which their genetic background or history had indicated might occur.

Amniocentesis is not done before the fifteenth or sixteenth week of pregnancy, in order to allow time for enough amniotic fluid to develop. If you do decide to proceed, you will find it a rather simple, painless, and brief process. It can be somewhat expensive, usually costing several hundred dollars. (Some of the cost may be covered by health insurance.) It takes about as much time to have the fluid sample drawn as you would spend in a usual doctor's office visit. A second visit might be necessary for hearing the results and the interpretation, unless the findings confirm that there are no problems.

You would probably have amniocentesis done in a hospital examining room on an outpatient basis, although it is sometimes carried out in a doctor's office. You lie on your back on an examining table with your abdomen unclothed and draped. The procedure involves the use of a hypodermic needle much like one used to take blood samples from a vein in your arm. An ultrasound scan is made, in order to guide the needle so that it does not touch either the fetus or the placenta. (You might ask to have the ultrasound equipment turned off as soon as guidance of the needle is finished, in order to avoid unnecessary exposure.)

A local anesthetic is usually given at the point on your abdomen selected as the site for inserting the needle. About 10 to 20 cubic centimeters (a few teaspoonfuls) of amniotic fluid are drawn out into the syringe. The procedure feels much the same as having a sizable blood specimen taken from your arm.

Analysis of the fluid sample requires two to three weeks. The sample contains body cells from the fetus, which are grown in tissue cultures in a medical laboratory and then examined under a microscope. (In some cases, the cell cultures fail to develop and the pregnant woman must have a second fluid sample drawn a few weeks after the first.)

The analysis determines accurately whether a fetus does or does not have any one of about one hundred different genetic disorders. Authorities on genetic counseling in pregnancy note that only about 1 in 10 pregnant women who might benefit from amniocentesis actually have the procedure done. Authorities also observe that the procedure can have the effect of reducing rather than increasing the number of decisions to have an abortion.

A determination of the sex of the unborn baby may be a welcome by-product of amniocentesis. Clearly, that purpose alone is not worth the risk of infection, miscarriage, or hemorrhage. Interestingly, some parents ask not to be told the sex because they prefer to learn at birth.

An Alternative Test for Birth Defects

A chorionic villus biopsy may be recommended as an alternative to amniocentesis as a test for birth defects. This is an experimental technique attracting increasingly wide interest because it promises to have several advantages over amniocentesis. One main advantage is that it can be made early in pregnancy, in about the tenth week, rather than the fifteenth or sixteenth week.

No amniotic fluid is removed. Instead, under the guidance of high-resolution ultrasound, a catheter is inserted without any incision or puncture, through the vagina and cervix and on into the uterus. The catheter is then used to painlessly clip or suction a tiny sample of the tissue on the outside of the developing fetal sac. This tissue consists largely of chorionic villi—threadlike protrusions which seem to help the sac develop a thick, spongy attachment to the wall of the uterus.

The catheter is then withdrawn and the fetal tissue sample is tested for evidence showing that the fetus does or does not have specific birth defects. Although this procedure is often described as painless, the necessary stabilization of the cervix and passage of instruments may be an uncomfortable experience.

If the chorionic villus biopsy technique is suggested, discuss the possible risks in detail with your care-giver. The technique can expose you to possible infection or miscarriage, and can expose the fetus to injury. It also involves possible long-term injury from exposure to ultrasound emissions. Benefits can include early findings on the fetus's imperfections, if any. However, it is in the experimental stage.

Deciding on Electronic Fetal Monitoring

You might be advised to have diagnoses made with another type of technology—electronic fetal monitoring (EFM). Its use might be recommended only in the last trimester or last few weeks of pregnancy.

In essence, health-care professionals use EFM to see how the heartbeat rate of the fetus responds to its own movements and to contractions of the mother's uterus. These responses indicate whether the placenta and fetal circulatory system, and also the fetal nervous system, are working well. If they are not working well, the fetus is probably in danger. Such early indications of danger may signal the health-care professional to recommend an early delivery by cesarean section.

Your health-care professional is not likely to suggest EFM if you are one of the large majority of expectant mothers clearly due to have a normal, low-risk childbirth. EFM is used to check on the health of the fetus only if some condition indicating potentially higher risk has appeared, such as:

- You are over 35 or 40 and are having your first baby, or are over age 45 and having a baby beyond your first.
- You have a serious health difficulty like a cardiac disease or diabetes.
- You have had an abnormal complication in a previous pregnancy.
- You are having complications in your current pregnancy.
- Your labor is overdue.

If one of these conditions fits your case, your health-care professional might advise you to have a diagnosis by EFM late in your pregnancy in conjunction with one or both of the following tests.

Nonstress Test

A nonstress test (NST) might be suggested in the last two or three months if you appear to be having a high-risk pregnancy for any of the first four reasons above. Some obstetricians think it important in their management of a high-risk pregnancy to give an NST test every week starting as early as the last two months before labor.

Or you might be advised to have an NST test very late in your pregnancy for the fifth reason—a labor apparently overdue by two weeks or more.

The NST test can be made in a doctor's office, clinic, or hospital. You lie down on an examining table, with your abdomen unclothed and draped, and a flat instrument about the size and weight of a wallet is loosely strapped over the location on your abdomen where the fetal heartbeat can be heard best. This device simply picks up the sounds of your baby's heartbeat and transmits them to the monitor for recording.

During the test you will probably be able to watch the main monitor unit—a box of electronic apparatus about the size of a small suitcase. Across the front are switches, dials, and indicator lights. An inset in the front carries a roll of graph paper on which the device's tracing pens and other internal markers record the inputs.

One of these pens traces the fetal heartbeat on the paper. Normally, an unborn baby has a heartbeat rate ranging from about 120 to 160 beats a minute; the rate can vary at times to as low as 100 or as high as 180 a minute without giving cause for concern. (Your own adult pulse rate at rest probably runs around 70 to 75 a minute, incidentally.)

For the nonstress test you will be given a monitor unit cable to hold. Once the test has begun, you'll be asked to press the button on the end of the cable every time you feel the fetus move inside you. An arrow or other clear marking will be printed on the graph each time you push the button.

With a fetus whose circulatory and nervous systems are developing well, the heartbeat rate varies from instant to instant as its activities and those of its mother change. A noticeable movement by the healthy fetus is followed by an increase in heartbeat rate. The nonstress test records and measures such increases. In the accepted view, NST results are normal or properly "reactive" if two or more movements by the fetus within twenty minutes are followed promptly by minimum increases of fifteen heartbeats a minute for at least fifteen seconds.

If a nonstress test produces patterns indicating "nonreactive" or negative results—patterns that do not show sufficient increases in the heartbeat rate of the fetus—a second type of EFM test will usually be made in order to provide more conclusive findings about fetal health. This is the contraction stress test (CST). In professional experience, relatively few women who are given the NST—perhaps on the order of 1 out of 10—have nonreactive results and thus seem to need the CST.

Oxytocin Challenge Test, or Contraction Stress Test

The OCT/CST is given in much the same way as the NST, with three main differences:

1. You will not be given a button to push when you feel a fetal movement.

2. In addition to the flat, wallet-size instrument used to pick up the fetal heartbeat, a second similar instrument is strapped higher on the abdomen, near the top of the uterus. It is used to pick up and transmit the contractions of the uterus. Called a tocotransducer, it works essentially by detecting changes in the surface of your abdomen as your uterus contracts.

3. A glandular secretion called oxytocin is used to stimulate your uterus to mild contractions (they stop without going on to begin actual labor and delivery). Oxytocin is usually given by intravenous (IV) injection through a vein in the wrist.

The OCT/CST test measures the effect of uterine contractions on the heartbeat rate of the fetus. Reliable results call for recording the effect of at least three contractions within a ten-minute period, each lasting about forty seconds. Some women have mild prelabor contractions in the last few weeks of pregnancy that start and stop spontaneously at irregular times. These "Braxton-Hicks" contractions may suffice for an OCT/CST test. If so, an oxytocin IV would not be used.

Stimulation of the nipples causes the pituitary gland to produce your body's own oxytocin, which in turn sets off contractions of the uterus. In the last weeks of pregnancy you should be able to notice that contractions start soon after you begin massaging your nipples. Some health-care professionals use such nipple stimulation to produce the contractions for an OCT/CST instead of giving oxytocin intravenously.

But should you require an IV to stimulate the needed contractions, a dilute solution of oxytocin will be used, and its flow will be carefully controlled to stop the contractions before you go into labor.

Your OCT/CST test results are judged according to the way in which the contractions affect the heartbeat rate of the fetus. The results might indicate that everything seems fine. But if the placenta is not functioning well and the fetus is compromised during contractions, these conditions would be indicated in the penline patterns produced in the test. These findings, combined with other indications, might result in a recommendation that you have a delivery very soon by cesarean section.

If labor is overdue by three weeks or more, induced labor may be recommended. In pregnancies that continue past the forty-second week, the placenta has aged and can become less effective in transporting nourishment, thereby seriously affecting the well-being of the fetus. Prompt delivery by induction or cesarean section is thought advisable if tests show fetal distress.

Your care-giver will probably elect *not* to do an OCT/CST test if any of the following conditions apply (because the test might begin premature labor or lead to other complications):

• You have had a premature labor in the past (or your present condition gives signs of possible premature labor.

• The amniotic sac has broken well before your due date.

• You have had a past cesarean section with an incision high on your uterus (rather than a low, transverse incision).

• You have bleeding from the vagina for a cause not yet determined.

• You have a complication involving the placenta (such as abruptio placentae, in which the placenta has begun to separate from the wall of the uterus before labor; or placenta previa, in which the placenta is located at the bottom of the uterus, blocking the cervical canal).

As with other types of advanced technologic methods, electronic fetal monitoring should be done only if clearly justified by the evidence. The main risk with the two tests is exposure of your unborn baby to ultrasound waves, about which a great deal remains to be learned. You should avoid even any possible harm unless it is outweighed by compelling concrete evidence of possible serious danger to your unborn baby or yourself.

7

Middle Pregnancy: The Second Trimester

The mid-trimester of pregnancy is for most women a time of never feeling better. Early discomforts have gone and the baby is not yet weighty or large enough to cause pressure or tire you, as it may in the last trimester.

Third Month (The Fourteenth Week) of Pregnancy

Your uterus will now be large enough to make your lower abdomen protrude. It will have grown to an extent that you'll probably be able to see, and also to gently feel with your fingertips through your abdominal wall.

Your baby will weigh around 3 or 4 ounces—that is, up to about a quarter-pound. As you can see in Figure 7.1, the placenta will be well developed (the spongy mass to the upper right of the fetus). This is the remarkable structure through which your system supplies all the food and oxygen for the baby. It is normally located on the rear or front wall of the uterus (rather than on its right or left wall).

Even this early, your baby will start exercising the muscles to be used later in such vital functions as sucking and breathing. By the sixteenth to nineteenth week, you are likely to feel the first movements of the fetus, called quickening. At the start, these are quite faint. They feel like soft fluttering, as if being made by something as delicate as the wings of a butterfly.

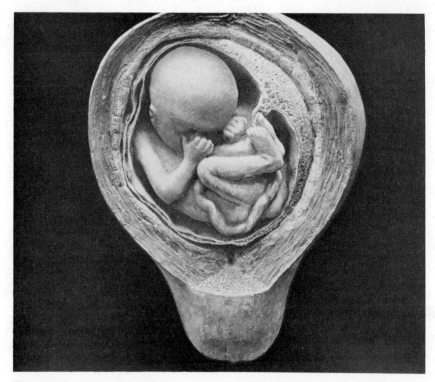

Figure 7.1. Fourteenth week

The Fifth Month

Very rapid growth during these weeks will bring the baby's length up to about 10 inches by the twenty-second week, or the end of the fifth month.

How the fetus lodges within your uterus (and how the uterus in turn lodges among your internal organs) is illustrated in Figure 7.2, a cross-sectional view of the expectant mother's trunk at about this time. The small and large intestine, stomach, liver, and other organs in the abdominal cavity have begun to be displaced upward in a gradual natural adjustment. The top of the uterus, or fundus, can be felt at about the level of the mother's navel.

Continued rising of the uterus in the abdominal cavity will relieve the pressure on the bladder (directly below the neck and head of the fetus in Figure 7.2) in the coming weeks. That in turn will reduce the need to empty the bladder often.

The same upward rise will cause the abdominal organs to push

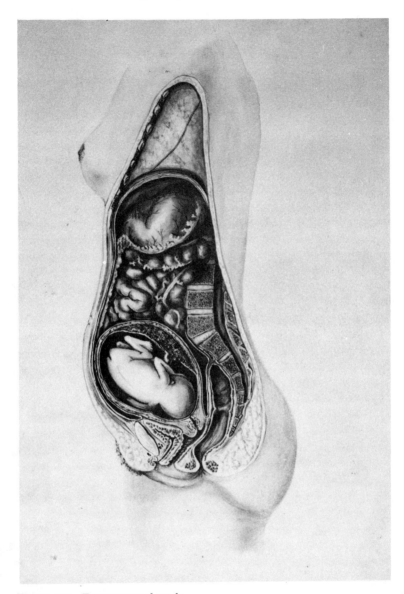

Figure 7.2. Twenty-second week

on the diaphragm at the top of the abdominal cavity, making it curve upward. This somewhat reduces the space available above the diaphragm for lung expansion. Less lung space, plus the breathing you are doing for the baby, may lead to a sensation of shortness of breath. Both factors warrant your decreasing your physical activity.

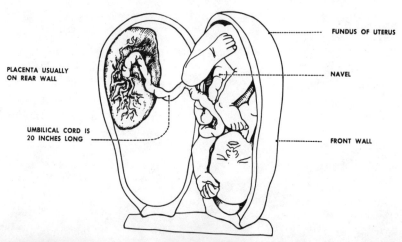

PLACENTA USUALLY
ON REAR WALL

FUNDUS OF UTERUS

NAVEL

UMBILICAL CORD IS
20 INCHES LONG

FRONT WALL

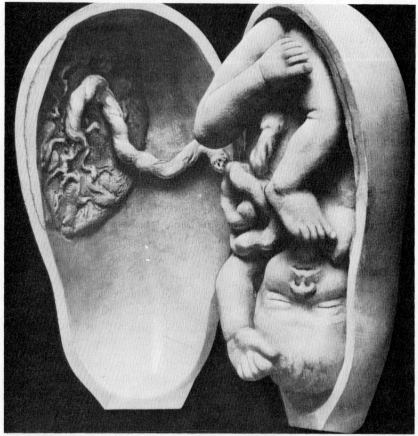

Figure 7.3. Twenty-eighth week

The Sixth Month

Your baby will have developed dramatically by the end of the sixth month; it looks almost fully formed. Hair may also have begun to grow on its eyebrows and head. You can see something of this in Figure 7.3. The photo and line drawing illustrate a fetus at about the twenty-eighth week, and display with special clarity the relationship of the uterus, placenta, and umbilical cord to the baby.

Besides looking nearly all formed, the baby at this time weighs as much as 2 or 2½ pounds. Nevertheless, many essential steps in the growth process remain ahead. For instance, the baby will triple his weight by the time of its birth.

In Figure 7.3, the uterus is pictured in front and rear halves for illustrative clarity, with the baby depicted in the front half. The placenta is the round structure on the rear wall. It's common for the placenta to be at the rear and the fetus in front, as shown here, but no special difficulty arises in normal pregnancies where the reverse happens to be true.

The umbilical cord between the placenta and fetus runs an ample 20 inches long to provide slack for movement by the baby. The cord rests comfortably between the placenta and the baby.

Handling Your Body for Comfort

Through these middle months when your uterus and the baby are rapidly growing much larger and heavier, you should adjust the ways in which you perform everyday actions like lifting, lying down, and getting up. This will make these movements easier and will protect you from muscle strains.

Standing, Walking, and Climbing Stairs

Using good posture while standing, walking, and going up stairs can do a great deal to head off fatigue and sore muscles.

Figure 7.4 illustrates the way to stand most comfortably as your unborn baby grows larger:

- Keep your feet spread somewhat apart, just about parallel, and with your weight balanced equally between them. Keep your legs straight but without tensing your knees.
- Hold your abdominal wall comfortably firm, pulling it in and up, while also holding your buttock muscles firm and tucking them down. (See pages 140–147 for helpful exercises.)

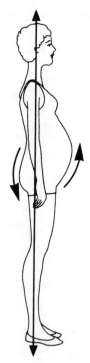

Figure 7.4. Good standing posture

- Let the weight of the fetus be carried by your hip bones, not by your abdominal wall. Women who lean back to compensate for the forward bulge are described as displaying "the pride of pregnancy." Walking behind such women, you can tell that they are "great with child." But this posture is very hard on the skeleton and its supporting muscles, and should be avoided. Instead, cradle the baby in your bony pelvic "girdle."

- Hold this posture when carrying packages. Use shopping bags with handles or a cart for any heavy packages, rather than letting them throw you off balance. When using a broom or similar tool, put one foot forward and out to the side to keep your balance.

Figure 7.5 shows how to handle yourself when going up steps:

- Start with the good standing posture just portrayed.
- Take hold of the railing, if there is one, and firmly place your full foot rather than just your toes on each step.

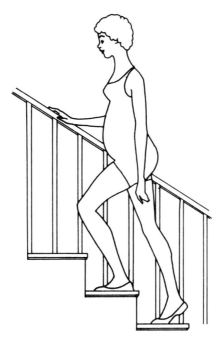

Figure 7.5. Climbing stairs

- Use your leg muscles to lift you without leaning forward and putting a strain on your back muscles.
- Breathe deeply and regularly as you climb; pause and breathe enough times at each landing to catch your breath if you're going up more than one flight.

In late pregnancy, when your abdomen protrudes, turn your body slightly sideways so you can see each step clearly before putting your foot on it.

Stooping and Lifting

As your pregnancy advances, you should be increasingly careful about the way you stoop down and lift things.

Figure 7.6 depicts the way to get at things near or on the floor. Bending over from the waist strains your back muscles. Instead, do this:

- Bend your knees and sink down to a crouching or squatting position, keeping your back straight and head erect.

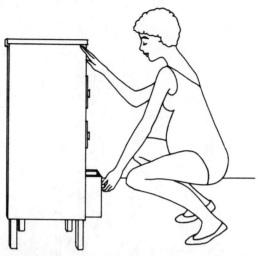

Figure 7.6. Stoop down by crouching—not by bending over

- Keep your balance by placing your feet and knees wide apart while continuing to hold your back straight.

If you can avoid it, don't lift anything heavy. But when you must lift, proceed as shown in Figure 7.7. The sequence should go as follows:

1. Put one foot forward, and lower your body slowly until your weight is resting on the other knee. Steady yourself by grasping solid furniture if available.
2. Gather the child or object close to you, and rise by using the muscles of your forward leg rather than your back muscles. Use the toes of your rear foot for balance and to push as you rise.
3. Keep your back upright, not bent over, as you lift and rise.

Rather than lifting little children, use other methods when feasible. Sit down on a chair and have the toddler climb up onto your lap, for instance. Or have the child climb a stepstool while you stand beside for safety, and then pick up the child from the stool.

Lying Down and Getting Up

Even lying in bed can be made far more comfortable by certain techniques. Using a second pillow under your head may help relieve discomfort from such sources as shortness of breath, lower back pain,

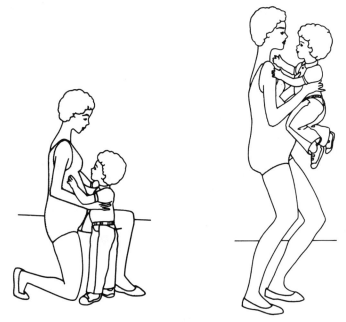

Figure 7.7. Avoid lifting—but when you must, lift this way

or pressure on the ribs. Placing the added pillow the long way, so that it extends under your shoulders, can help prevent neck strain.

Your legs may relax more if you put a folded blanket or a pillow under your thighs. However, don't put such supports behind your knees (placing them there can reduce the circulation of blood to your lower legs). Letting your legs and feet roll outward can be restful. Moving each leg in outward rolls like this can help ease lower back pain.

One major precaution: do not lie flat on your back for any length of time in your pregnancy. The heavy weight of the uterus in this position can squeeze on major blood vessels, resulting in lowered blood pressure and a feeling of faintness. The lower illustration in Figure 7.8 shows a lying-down variation that is useful in later pregnancy.

A position many expectant mothers find increasingly comfortable late in pregnancy is shown in Figure 7.9. It is also found to be helpful for short time spans during labor. This is the closest you would come to a chest-down position late in pregnancy. Lie on either side (whichever is more comfortable) and place one or two pillows diagonally under your head, upper shoulder, and upper breast; let your enlarged abdomen rest on the bed, possibly with a folded towel or small pillow underneath for support; put a pillow under the knee of your upper leg if it makes your back or your abdomen feel more comfortable.

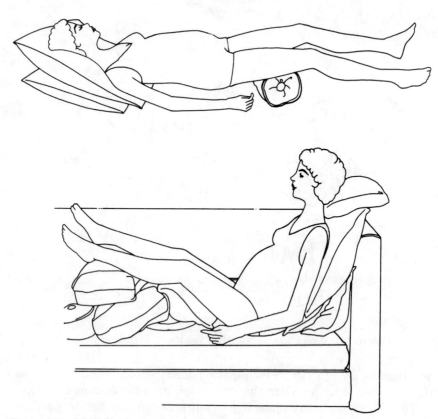

Figure 7.8. Prop your back for comfort when lying down

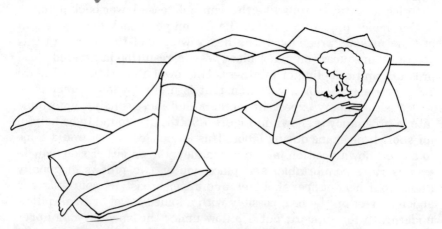

Figure 7.9. First side-lying position for advanced pregnancy and labor

94

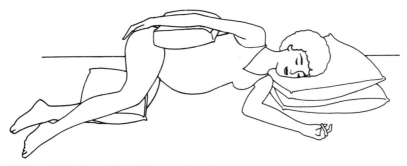

Figure 7.10. Second side-lying position for pregnancy and labor

Another side position is shown in Figure 7.10: Lie on the side that's most comfortable for you, and put one or two pillows under your head (but not under your shoulder) as needed for height. Bend your knees slightly and keep them together; you might place a small pillow or folded towel between your legs if you are more comfortable that way.

Should the arm you're lying on start tingling and getting numb, put a rolled blanket or folded pillow lengthwise against your back. Leaning gently against it should relieve the pressure on your arm.

To get out of bed easily and safely, move to the side-lying position shown in Figure 7.11 (if you are not already in that position), turning your hips and shoulders at the same time; place the hand of your upper arm so that it can push flat against the bed; and slide your knees and feet so that they're right on the edge of the bed. Push with your arms to rise slowly while you swing your lower legs down over the side of the bed. Pause for a short time while sitting on the edge of the bed, taking several deep breaths before you stand up. Changes in position can cause lightheadedness as your circulatory system adapts.

Emotional Developments in Middle Pregnancy

Compared to the feelings in early pregnancy, expectant mothers in the middle three months typically experience greater comfort, energy, and confidence. Such a sense of well-being develops as you become better adjusted both physically and emotionally to being pregnant. Physically, the nausea experienced by some women often goes away after the third month of pregnancy. The lifting of the uterus, as the fetus grows, eases the pressure on the bladder and thereby relieves the need to urinate frequently.

With increasing adaptation of your system to pregnancy, you may

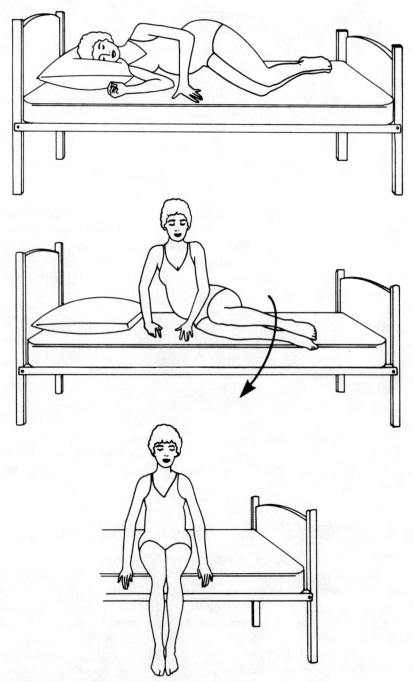

Figure 7.11. Getting out of bed without strain throughout pregnancy

feel less tired and much more energetic after the third month. Many women find they never felt better nor looked lovelier than in these middle months, when their whole being seems to be working with far more zest than ever before.

Your excitement and wonder will probably grow as you feel and hear your baby more and more during these middle months. At some time in the late fourth or early fifth month, you will probably start to feel the baby bumping you at times with a kick or a shifted arm. And around this time you and your partner may well start listening to your baby's heartbeat with a stethoscope while you are carrying out a health checkup with the professional providing your prenatal care.

At around the sixth month you might start to notice times of increasingly lively movement by your baby. These are likely to come when you are resting, perhaps just before going off to sleep. The baby finds it easier to move when you're still and when your abdominal wall is relaxed. You may even see your abdomen bulge out with the poke of a tiny foot or elbow when you're lying quietly and baby is having an active time. You can communicate with your fetus, too, pushing gently on your abdomen and feeling a responsive movement. When you are active during the day, though, it often seems that the baby is rocked by your movements and less active.

If your experience is like that of quite a few expectant parents, you and your partner may grow closer and more thoughtful of each other as your unborn baby becomes ever more real, responsive, and familiar. Your ties as a couple can deepen and broaden with the new cares and feelings of pregnancy. Picking out prenatal classes that you can both attend is one of many new experiences that may draw you together. And in general, you'll probably have a growing sense of doing something important with your lives.

8

The Third Trimester

Anticipation and even some impatience build through the last trimester, which completes the growth of your baby and culminates in birth.

The Eighth Month

You and your baby will both have been growing at almost the most rapid rate of your entire pregnancy in the weeks before the thirty-sixth week, or the end of the eighth month. The baby will be quite large by this time, as shown in Figure 8.1. She or he will probably weigh 6 to 7 pounds and measure (if outstretched) about 18 inches long.

As for your own weight, you will very likely have put on just about all the weight you'll be gaining while pregnant. The baby may gain another pound or so in the remaining month; you might or might not add a little more weight yourself.

However, you should definitely not grow heavier at anything like the fast rate of prior weeks, which was necessary for healthy growth of the baby. At that fast rate you probably put on something like one-fourth of your total weight gain in the seventh month alone.

Your baby, though able to move actively and strongly at this point, is constricted in space. You may be really jolted by a kick or prod. A kick in the direction of your ribs may be so sharp at times that it makes you gasp. You may also be surprised to feel the baby sometimes give a steady series of rhythmic twitches. These are hiccups, caused

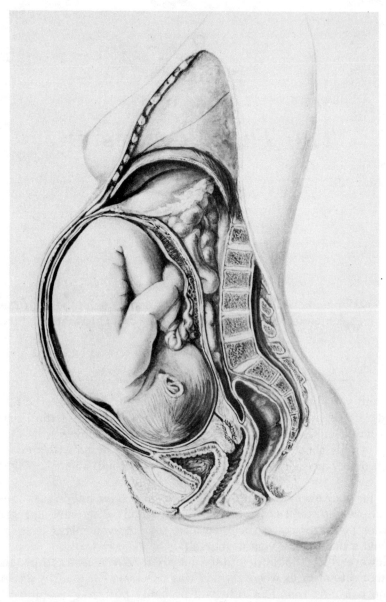

Figure 8.1. Eighth month

by the immaturity of its nervous system and spasms in the phrenic nerve, which activates the diaphragm.

By this time your baby can open its eyes and can see the difference between light and dark; presumably it's aware of a warm red glow when you're out in the bright sunlight and wearing thin clothes. It also hears, and jumps suddenly with the "startle reaction" when surprised by a loud noise. The soft prenatal fuzz called lanugo that had covered its skin is shedding off, and the creamy whitish vernix, also protecting its skin, is diminishing as it dissolves in the amniotic fluid.

In addition, by this time your baby will probably have shifted into the head-down position in which it will remain through birth. The majority of babies do take such a position in the uterus. However, a small proportion (about 3 percent) take a "breech" position, with the buttocks or feet first, and a still smaller proportion get into various kinds of sideways positions. The positions other than head-down need careful monitoring through the last weeks of pregnancy and on into labor.

In your own system, as indicated in Figure 8.1, the uterus will grow to occupy most of the abdominal cavity and will leave your stomach, liver, and intestines crowded together. You may consequently find it better to shift to eating smaller and more frequent meals. You can also see in Figure 8.1 how the top, or fundus, of the uterus will reach its maximum height in about the thirty-sixth week. The fundus will extend up to just under your breastbone, or sternum.

Those mild Braxton-Hicks contractions of the uterus, which you have probably felt from time to time for some weeks already, should be occurring more often and more noticeably at this point. These are sometimes called practice or rehearsal contractions; they are spontaneous waves of tightening of the uterine wall, and may be felt occasionally from the fifth or sixth month on.

You will also be likely to feel rather sharp twinges in your left or right side. These are caused by sudden pulls on the large vertical round ligaments supporting the uterus (as illustrated earlier, in Figure 5.2).

Your feet and wrists may exhibit some swelling from increased retention of fluid late in pregnancy. Moderate fluid buildup like this is normal and provides potentially valuable protection during childbirth; hot weather may intensify the buildup.

Your nipples may already have begun to exhibit an occasional slight flow of a thick yellowish liquid. This is colostrum, which precedes the supply of breast milk and is a highly nutritious substance for the baby to consume right after birth. Hormonal changes in your system may also result in more vaginal lubrication than you usually have, and may similarly give rise to some swelling and congestion of your nasal membranes.

You might also often feel heavy, as well as drowsy and languid. If you feel like it, take your time in getting about and get more rest than usual, in naps and nighttime sleep. You really are carrying a very substantial extra load, which uses a large part of your strength and energy.

The Ninth Month

Your baby will now have grown still larger, some 7 pounds in weight and 20 inches in length. The baby may also have completed the downward shift called lightening or dropping, and the head may be "engaged." You can see this portrayed in Figure 8.2.

As illustrated there (and discussed in Chapter 13), lightening represents a movement of the baby downward, with its head extending well into the cradle of the pelvic bones. Lightening usually takes place almost unnoticeably over a period of time in the last few weeks of pregnancy; on occasion, it can happen noticeably. With it occur a number of important internal changes easily seen by comparing Figures 8.2 and 8.1.

The cervix is shorter but still closed. The abdomen protrudes to the greatest extent in pregnancy. Pressure will have eased, creating space in the upper abdomen, so you will feel less constriction in breathing.

Pressure will have increased, however, in your lower abdomen. Less room for your bladder will make you urinate more frequently, as in the first trimester. Similarly, less room for the rectum might contribute to some constipation. And the pressure of the baby's head and weight in your lower groin can make your legs ache from time to time.

You will probably be able to feel the baby making a number of the same movements it will perform after it's born. For instance, you may notice a fast back-and-forth kind of motion. That's likely to be the baby's head turning as it searches to retrieve a thumb on which it has been sucking.

Emotional Developments Near Pregnancy's End

Swings in Emotion

Go easy on yourself in these last few weeks. You're approaching a major experience in your life, a milestone. Expect that your emotions may swing widely from great joy and elation to fretful impatience or some uncertainty, worry, and gloom.

Ease yourself out of low spots or annoyances if they occur:

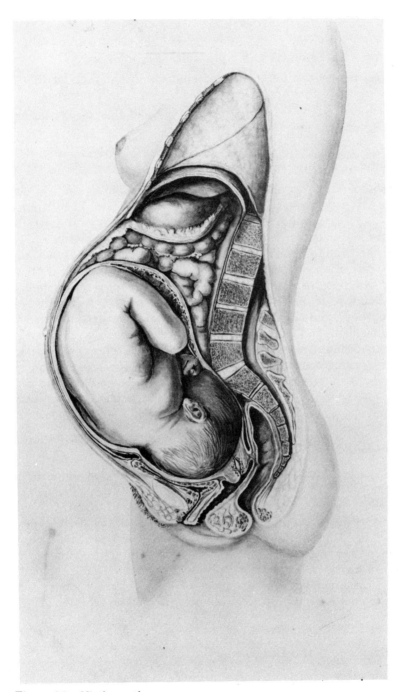

Figure 8.2. Ninth month

- Talk to your partner and supportive friends.
- Keep involved in work, interests, and activities you enjoy insofar as possible, rather than simply waiting in idleness.
- Reassure yourself that marked changes in emotions at this time are quite normal and that the negative ones will soon pass.
- Busy yourself with getting your home and the baby's equipment and clothes ready.

Fatigue

It is important to guard against physical weakness and fatigue in these last few weeks. Keep up your nutritious diet. Take particular care to avoid anemia (by including enough iron in your diet). If you always feel tired, have your blood hemoglobin level checked.

Sheer tiredness might also bother you at this time. If it does, use the best antidote: rest. Your system is doing a great deal of work, even when you're sitting still. Get as much more rest, through naps and hours of nighttime sleep, as you may need to feel fully rested.

Depression and fear sometimes trouble women late in pregnancy. Dreams about the baby's health can be recurrent. Teachers and students in prenatal classes, and class sessions themselves, can be effective in countering such anxious feelings. Turn to the people you chose for emotional support—they can really help bolster you up. Should your mood persist despite your efforts to relieve it, ask the professional providing your prenatal health care for further suggestions.

"Nest-Building"

In the days before labor starts, you may get sudden impulses—and the energy—to bustle through certain ambitious tasks. Some women feel they simply must paint and redecorate a bedroom. Others are compelled to do a complete whirlwind housecleaning. Still others feel moved to shop for masses of reserve groceries and household supplies.

Such unexpected surges of purpose and vitality are commonly experienced, but as yet there is no generally accepted scientific explanation. We can assume that they stem from some ancient evolutionary instinct to carry out a kind of nest-building in preparation for the arrival of our young.

Anxiety about the Due Date

Quite a lot of impatience and annoyance in these last weeks and days of pregnancy often results from a natural but inescapable fact: the exact arrival date of the baby continues to be uncertain. These emotions can be intense for some expectant parents; you can avoid them almost completely by taking a few simple precautions, which consist largely of remembering the following facts:

- *Your baby may arrive two weeks or more before the due date.* The due date around which you've been planning all through pregnancy is only a "best guess," even if a professional helped you derive it. In fact, some 30 out of every 100 babies arrive early, and only about 5 out of every 100 actually arrive exactly on schedule.

- *Your baby may arrive ten days to two weeks after the due date.* Most babies start life later than forecast—as many as 65 out of every 100. About 10 out of every 100 babies are born more than ten days past their due dates.

Think of your due date as only a broad guess, and assume that your baby can arrive at any time from two weeks before to two weeks later. Plan to complete all your essential preparations two weeks before the due date, and map out activities that can keep you interested and occupied for as long as two weeks after that date. And except for anyone who will be coming to help you on your return home, give family and friends a date which is two to three weeks beyond the calculated due date, so that you will not be bothered by their inquiries should your baby be delayed. Let them be pleasantly surprised when you call first, with word of the baby's arrival.

9

⌢‿⠙⠉⠄⠌

Prenatal Care and
Types of Childbirth:
Making the Decisions

You need to understand that there is no such thing as risk-free child-birth. Making decisions about your prenatal and birth care, such as the care-provider, setting for birth, use of drugs and technology, is really selecting the package of risks most acceptable to you.

Good prenatal care begins well before conception. It's not called prenatal care then, of course, but the way a young woman has taken care of herself bears on her ability to conceive a healthy baby, nourish it well, and give birth. The way a mother feeds her infant daughter can help ensure healthy grandchildren. And the importance of healthy sperm is now recognized, too, so males must be included in the effort to ensure a healthy population. Teach your children early that once they arrive at a time in their lives when pregnancy is possible, it is wise to start to collect information on available maternity services.

Preferably before you become pregnant, but surely at some point early in pregnancy, investigate your options. The sooner you begin, the sooner you can enjoy the reassurance of working with experts you trust. Physicians and nurse-midwives should welcome your inquiries even though you may not yet be pregnant, and you should also be able to tour birth facilities.

The Alternatives for Childbirth

There are five basic "styles" of childbirth:

1. Home birth—nonprofessionally supervised (*NOT* recommended),
2. Home birth—professionally supervised,

3. Birth centers or childbearing centers (out-of-hospital),

4. Humanized hospital birth, including birth rooms and in-hospital alternative birth centers, and

5. Conventional hospital birth.

The first three options are suitable only when a normal birth is expected. They also require your active involvement, as does the fourth possibility, if yours is a low-risk pregnancy. The fifth choice functions best for a normal birth when you are more passive in nature, or for a complicated or multiple birth. However, even an at-risk situation might not require a conventional hospital approach. Birth rooms and in-hospital alternative birth centers often represent an attempt on the part of care-providers to humanize birth as much as possible even for those at risk. For example, with the newer techniques of monitoring and controlling blood sugar levels in pregnant diabetic women, a participatory vaginal birth is becoming more and more possible, but the hospital is still the preferred setting. In some instances, birth rooms and alternative birth centers in-hospital do not represent a "people change," but merely one of design and decoration. For this reason, it is very important for you to meet the people who will be caring for you as you look at services.

Investigate these options carefully, because the one you choose also determines to a large extent the type of practitioner you will engage for your maternity health care and the type of prenatal education you will undertake. Expectant parents often find it very hard to shift to another approach or care-giver once their initial choice has been made.

Keep in mind the fact that, just as no one can guarantee you a perfect, healthy baby, no alternative is entirely risk-free—not even birth in the world's most advanced hospital. After you are fully informed, you can decide which risks you are willing to take and which approach to childbirth is most reassuring and appropriate for you.

Home Birth

Today many expectant parents representing all social backgrounds are considering having labor and delivery right in their own homes. Their numbers have continued to increase slowly but steadily in recent years, despite difficulties in locating qualified care-providers willing to attend home births.

Nonprofessionally supervised: This first alternative is also known as do-it-yourself home birth. It was the limitations and inherent risks of this type of birth which motivated the Maternity Center Association to establish the carefully planned and professionally staffed Childbearing Center, in order to provide a more acceptable option for those families who are so alienated from hospitals that they have left the health-care system completely.

In such a birth, you might be aided through labor and delivery by either an informally apprenticed, probably unlicensed, lay-midwife or by someone without any special preparation in maternity care, perhaps the baby's father or a woman relative or friend who has had babies herself.

Prenatal care should of course always be available but may not be with this type of arrangement, and there may or may not be any provision for transferring you and/or your new baby to a hospital should special problems develop.

This birth alternative has the decisive disadvantage of risks that are unmanageable. Our conclusion for this alternative is therefore: **not recommended.**

Professionally supervised: You could, however, reasonably consider professionally supervised home birth for a normal or low-risk birth. In this option, your health care through pregnancy and labor is provided by a formally prepared practitioner licensed to provide maternity services:

- a physician (an M.D. or D.O. functioning either as a general practitioner or as a specialist in obstetrics),
- a certified nurse-midwife (C.N.M.),
- a licensed lay-midwife (in a state that licenses lay-midwives; always inform yourself as to what is required for the license—the maternal and child health division of your state health department can help you), or
- other practitioners licensed to attend birth (see page 6).

In this alternative, your practitioner's training and education also enables him or her to provide your prenatal and postpartum care (care after the birth) and to arrange for expert consultation and care within the hospital system if needed. The practitioner should be qualified to help you determine what low-risk and higher-risk conditions are probable in your case.

This type of home birth can help you realize almost all the values associated with family-centered childbearing:

- *Sharing by the couple:* the companionship, support, and participation of the partner and all other family members in the birth.

- *Focus on health:* the experience of birth as a healthy physiological process rather than a pathological one.
- *Greater control over the conditions of birth:* for families who recognize that the primary responsibility for health rests with themselves, an opportunity to exercise that responsibility by having the birth at home.
- *Greater physical and emotional strength:* a total setting of surroundings, people, and attitudes that tends to maximize both the emotional and the physiological strengths of the childbearing parents.
- *Avoidance of possible drawbacks of hospital birth:* including various features of conventional hospital birth which the couple may find disagreeable, frightening, or even hazardous (separation of the mother from loved ones and from the newborn, chemical and technologic intervention in the birth process, possibly needless cesarean surgery, the risk of hospital-generated infection, and high hospital costs).

On the other hand, these are disadvantages to professionally supervised home birth:

- *Difficulties in arranging hospital backup:* Many hospitals are fearful of receiving women or infants from a home birth and may refuse to agree in advance to accept a transfer; this factor increases home-birth hazards.
- *Scarcity of professionals to help with home birth:* The possible hazards and other difficulties connected with home birth—including opposition from colleagues—lead many qualified professionals to decide against being involved. As a result, couples interested in home birth may not find any professionals willing to assist them.
- *Lack of coverage by health insurance:* Some families are deterred from home birth by the fact that the costs of maternity care at home may not be reimbursed by their health insurance carrier.
- *Scheduling problems:* A care-provider may have difficulty adjusting his or her work load to be present for a home birth.

Obviously home birth should be considered only by expectant parents for whom a low-risk, normal delivery can be responsibly diagnosed. Pregnancies that involve some degree of higher-than-normal risk in labor and delivery can be most predictably managed in a setting in which specialists and up-to-date technology are available.

Even careful predictions of low-risk deliveries can change. This happens only in a small percentage of cases, but when it does, it is very important that a system for transfer to a hospital be in place. On rare occasions, an emergency transfer will be necessary.

Some young families feel the need for home birth despite the drawbacks. It is a sad state of affairs when people do not trust health-care providers or the settings that the providers control. But many home-birth couples select that option because of this mistrust. They reason that the behavior of the providers will be more responsive in a setting that the family controls. They further believe that if unwelcome management in labor and birth should occur, it can be stopped by ordering the provider from the home.

The necessity for such an extreme remedy is to be avoided. One of the tenets of nurse-midwifery practice is its emphasis on genuine accommodation to the wishes of women and families in any setting, including the hospital, so long as those wishes are not in direct violation of principles of safety. But in the final analysis, decisions on which risks they will run are up to the families. All providers should see that families are fully and legally informed.

Problems in working out the scheduling aspects of providing home-birth maternity care act as a further limit on the numbers of professionals who offer such services. Although birth itself is the time that requires the most intensive professional attendance, your longer preceding labor is equally if not more important for professional evaluation and management. It can often happen in a maternity-care practice that two or more women will go into labor at about the same time. At such times an individual practitioner would find it difficult or impossible to monitor and guide each birth fully. It is for this reason that professionals providing maternity-care services through labor and delivery most commonly practice in groups. But very few groups offer services for home births.

Precautions to take: If you choose home birth with professional supervision, be certain to make the following preparations:

1. Be assured with reasonable certainty that you have a very good chance of experiencing a normal, low-risk birth, as evidenced by a thorough analysis of your medical history and that of your family, a complete physical examination, and continuing prenatal checkups and care.

2. Select as your care-giver during pregnancy and labor a person who has completed a formal program of instruction, who is legally permitted to practice, and whom you trust completely by reason of that person's personal qualities, experience, and capability.

3. Prepare for labor and delivery as thoroughly as possible, through parent classes, learning important exercises and breathing techniques for labor, and reading.

4. Identify or tentatively set alternative arrangements for hospital delivery in case complications should develop during pregnancy.

5. Try to make arrangements in advance for possible transfer to a hospital during labor and for the transportation it would require.

Throughout the world today, the home remains by far the most common setting for birth; more than 80 percent of all babies are born at home, notes Dr. Sylvia Feldman in *Choices in Childbirth*.[1] And throughout the past centuries, birth almost always took place at home. Only in this century in this and other developed countries did hospital birth become the predominant choice. It became so conventional that in America today, less than 1 percent of all births take place at home. Still, gradually increasing numbers of expectant parents have decided to try home birth in recent years.

In sum, though, for all its attractive features, home birth with the assistance of a recognized professional is still difficult to arrange. Even if it is available in your locale, it's hard to guarantee that you can be safely transferred to a hospital in case of emergency.

Birth at an Out-of-Hospital Birth Center

Having your labor and delivery at a birth center run independently rather than as part of a hospital can offer many of the advantages of home birth while avoiding some of its possible hazards.

If you are likely to have a low-risk labor and delivery you can elect to use a birth center, where your birth experience will be family-centered and should include all important safety precautions. You have a good chance of finding such a birth center in your own area. Since the opening of MCA's demonstration Childbearing Center in 1975, more than 140 out-of-hospital birth centers have been started, and new ones continue to be opened in all parts of the country. The number should grow in coming years, through the work of an organization called the National Association of Childbearing Centers, established by MCA to provide practical information to others wanting to open birth centers. NACC also works toward high standards of care among its member centers, based on the extensive operating experience of MCA's Childbearing Center and other centers like it. A program for accrediting birth centers is also in place.

Key features of a birth center: Major elements of maternity care at one of these out-of-hospital birth centers include:

- homelike rooms for labor and birth in facilities outside hospitals and administered under autonomous policies, but with permanent arrangements for hospital transfer backup when needed, and for medical specialist consultation;
- the desirable qualities of home birth (presence of family members, flexible routines, nonseparation of infants and parents, decisions made by the family with care-giver's advice, opportunity to have a voice in policy-making);
- care provided by a team of licensed practitioners;
- availability of certain technologic supports in the event of emergency; and
- early release to return home (normally within 12 hours), with follow-up care.

Other advantages of using a birth center include:

- *Professionally safe care:* Safe care by a qualified professional staff with advance arrangements for emergency hospital transfer if needed.
- *Healthy, conscious birth experience:* Experiencing childbirth as a normal, healthy event without anesthetics or routine pain medications (60 percent of women at birth centers give birth without local anesthetics or analgesics, although centers are equipped to administer them if needed).
- *Sharing by the couple:* If desired, having the emotional support of a partner and other immediate family members, including brothers and sisters of your new baby, sharing in the experience.
- *Avoidance of possible hospital birth drawbacks:* Use of a birth center precludes the same kinds of disagreeable, frightening, or routine features of conventional hospital birth that home birth avoids.
- *Cost:* Costs for a normal childbirth at a birth center are only 40 to 50 percent of the total costs for a normal childbirth in a hospital. There are a number of reasons for this: Birth centers use residential space (with minor adaptations) instead of expensive hospital space. In many, nurse-midwives provide the prenatal, intrapartum, and postpartum care; physicians consult and manage problems of complication or pathology if they arise. The emphasis on nonintervention

is cost-effective, since all machine and chemical modalities for patient care are costly. And prenatal parent classes in caring for newborns facilitate early discharge and allow for minimal professional supervision of after-care.

- *Reimbursement:* As insurers and purchasers of benefits become more aware of and knowledgeable about birth centers, reimbursement, usually at full fee, becomes more available. Some 170 insurers currently include birth-center care in their health insurance coverage.

- *Regulation:* At this writing, twenty-four states have adopted regulations to ensure sound standards for birth centers. Such regulations have resulted largely from guidelines adopted by the American Public Health Association with the assistance of the National Association of Childbearing Centers and its predecessor organization, the Cooperative Birth Center Network.

- *Accreditation:* Accreditation represents a step beyond licensure in furthering high quality care. The Commission on Accreditation established by NACC is supervising site visiting and review of birth centers based on accepted standards. The knowledge that a center is accredited can assist you in decision-making.

Now let's consider the possible disadvantages of using a birth center for your prenatal care and birth.

- *Takes much time and effort:* The birth center alternative requires a substantial amount of effort and time on the part of the pregnant woman and her support partner. They must attend weekly classes for six to twelve weeks, must both learn and practice exercises and techniques to use during labor, and must spend time studying reference and supplementary materials they get in class. Some expectant parents feel that they would prefer to leave all this to their care-provider and just do a bare minimum to prepare for labor and delivery.

- *Doesn't feel as safe as a hospital:* Some expectant parents do not wish to run the risk of emergency transfer and believe they would be more secure with the scientific technology of a hospital immediately at hand. Statistics showing that emergency transfers are rare and that birth centers are at the very least as safe as hospitals do not offset their feeling that a hospital is the safest place even for normal, low-risk childbirth.

- *Concern over possible transfer:* Some families fear having to move during labor from a birth center to a hospital that would not offer all the reassuring features of a center. So great is this concern for a few families that they would rather not chance the disappointment of a transfer.

The question of safety: Safety at a birth center is fostered by five considerations:

1. Orientation of interested parents to develop their understanding of the risks of childbearing in general and at the center specifically, so that they can make an informed and confident decision.
2. Physical screening of expectant parents to ensure that a low-risk birth can be predicted.
3. A qualified professional staff, with the director preferably a certified nurse-midwife (C.N.M.) or a physician who understands the low-tech/high-touch practice of midwifery; a qualified obstetrical consultant as director of medical affairs; enough additional C.N.M. staff members so that a C.N.M. will attend each birth with the aid of at least a second staff person (such as a trained midwife assistant); full obstetrical admitting privileges to the backup hospital, held by the center's medical affairs director, so that continuity of care is available to all families.
4. Emphasis on preventive care to forestall potential health problems in advance, with relevant physical examinations and regular monitoring of health throughout the pregnancy by both professionals and the expectant parents themselves, and with the provision of thoroughgoing prenatal classes, informal counseling, and informational materials for extensive parent education.
5. A planned system for transfer of the mother and/or infant to an acute-care hospital if indicated, and basic items of emergency equipment (including an infant transfer isolette, infant warmer, oxygen, resuscitation trays for mother and infant, oxygen, and intravenous fluids including blood-volume expander).

Some prospective parents interested in using a birth center view the centers' rigorous screening for low-risk birth as a disadvantage— if the screening excludes them. Although a proportion of persons cannot pass the screening, some can bring their health into eligible range by correcting such conditions as anemia or a weight problem (high or low) before becoming pregnant.

Humanized Hospital Birth

Hospitals providing what we term humanized birth have incorporated various features of family-centered childbirth in their maternity care.

Which features you actually find will vary widely from one hospital to another, according to overall policies and attitudes. Most hospitals will share certain factors that set them apart from birth centers:

- Prenatal care and education services are likely to be given at sites away from the place where you'll give birth and by persons who aren't part of the staff with you throughout labor.

- Labor and delivery may be carried out in what are still essentially surgical operating rooms rather than homelike birth rooms (though increasing numbers of hospitals are introducing such birth rooms and in-hospital birth centers). Use of surgical rooms will in turn require that you be moved from the labor to the delivery area.

- Children and family members other than the baby's father probably will not be allowed to visit you in the hospital during labor and just after you give birth.

- Labor and birth will likely occur near to or in the high-tension labor and delivery suite, restricting your freedom to walk around while you are in labor.

- Depersonalized hospital procedures and attitudes may intrude on your emotional experience at some points—such as routine application of technology (fetal electronic monitoring, for instance), when it may be neither needed nor wanted. Also, your baby may be kept from you for an observation period after the birth.

- You are considered a patient and have little control over the setting. Professionals have control.

- It is unlikely that a family member could prepare a meal for a celebration following the birth.

- There may be a reluctance to release you early to return home.

What you view as advantages and disadvantages of this type of alternative will depend on your preferences between the extremes of a free-standing birth center on the one hand and a conventional hospital birth on the other. In general, though, you can expect far less flexibility with what you want in your labor and birth experience at a hospital with many maternity patients than at a birth center serving far fewer families.

Features to look for: Interestingly, the recent growth of the out-of-hospital birth center has resulted in hospitals increasingly adapting their maternity floors to meet rising demand for more family-centered childbirth. The family-centered features you might look for in humanized hospital services include the:

- opportunity for family members in addition to the expectant father to remain with the mother during labor and delivery;
- opportunity for the mother to go through labor and delivery with no analgesia or anesthesia if she wishes and is able to do so;
- opportunity for a Leboyer birth, in which the new parents hold, comfort, and communicate with their new baby in a mutual emotional "bonding" (which is thought to be a very positive experience by many parents and maternity-care practitioners);
- provision of a well-developed nurse-midwifery service. By training and professional orientation, nurse-midwives often are able to devote more time and place more emphasis on fostering a family-centered birth than do many physicians attending birth. As a result, a strong nurse-midwifery service in a hospital usually reflects a special dedication in that hospital policy to family-centered birth experiences.

Family-centered birth features you might find less frequently, but which are worth seeking, include the opportunity to walk around and to take any position that feels comfortable during labor, "rooming-in" for the baby (whereby it stays in a crib in the mother's hospital room most of the time rather than in the nursery), extended visiting hours for the new father, and visiting hours for siblings, with preparatory classes.

Some typical birth-center practices are not likely to be found at hospitals offering humanized birth programs, such as having very young children in the next room or even in the same room attending the birth of their brother or sister, having one or two close relatives or friends other than the father present for the birth, and being able to take a shower soon after you've had the baby, or having your support partner cook some food for a family meal and just feeling at home in the surroundings in which your prenatal care was given.

Conventional Hospital Birth

You probably know at least something about conventional or traditional hospital childbirth from having visited close relatives or friends who have had their babies in hospitals. Basic elements of such conventional hospital birth include:

- isolation of the mother through many of the hours she spends in labor (possibly up to ten hours or more), not only from her husband or other support partner but also from any other close family members or friends;

- lack of a constant professional attendant during labor (nursing staff members often must leave to take care of more urgent tasks);
- lack of continuous presence during labor by the attending physician or obstetrician, except for brief periods when that professional checks on her progress;
- complete dependence of the mother on outside control: she is permitted to attempt nothing and is required to accept passively whatever is done to her, however frightened or distressed she may feel, and to follow directions without serious question;
- underlying alarm or foreboding that results from the surroundings of technologic medical apparatus and the commonly found detached, impersonal, "professional" attitudes of nurses and other hospital attendants;
- threatening, unnerving, and uncomfortable or painful procedures done as a matter of routine, including shaving the pubic area, giving an enema, starting an intravenous drip, and enforced bed rest;
- the routine administration of analgesics or anesthetics;
- isolation of the baby after birth from the mother and family; and
- continued management of the mother after the birth as a hospital patient not permitted to care for her new baby.

Arrangements and practices of conventional hospital birth are adapted for serious potential complications. They also reflect the assumption that pregnancy is an illness and childbirth, a surgical procedure. There may be advantages in such handling for expectant parents for whom complications seem likely, or for expectant parents who feel more secure in an approach like this. However, some authorities maintain that parents who are at risk of complicated birth are even more in need of the supportive aspects of family-centered care. New mothers and their partners need each other most when they have a sick or ill-formed baby.

Conventional hospital birth—a medical profile: To give further insight, here's a brief review of conventional hospital birth as often practiced:

- specialist-dominated, with routine intervention such as: amniotomy (artificial rupture of membranes), use of ultrasound and electronic monitors, Pitocin intensification of labor, analgesia and regional or general anesthesia, and intravenous fluids
- lithotomy position for birth (lying on one's back)
- separation of family members

- de-emphasis of childbirth education and breastfeeding
- high value placed on "benefits" of cesarean section
- assumption of consumer inability and lack of desire to participate in decision-making
- neonatal period also likely to be technologically conducted

How to Reach Sound Decisions about Prenatal Care and Birth

Looking at today's alternatives for childbirth in the light of medical and cultural perspectives may well clear up unconscious biases, and in turn help you to reach more satisfying decisions for your own child-bearing experience.

The Medical Perspective on Birthing

The predominant way to have a baby in America is by conventional hospital birth. We have been acculturated to it as the regular or "right" way, not only as the experience of people we know, but also in countless portrayals in TV, movies, novels, magazines, and newspapers. So familiar is it that many Americans aren't even aware of other approaches. Indeed, many observers feel that the institutionalization of childbirth is responsible for the improvement in maternal and infant outcomes and doubtless it does deserve some of the credit. Improved public health measures relating to nutrition, sanitation, and child spacing have also played a role.

Many of us assume that the use of advanced technology and the other common practices of conventional hospital birth are based on masses of scientific evidence. We take it for granted that the predominant way of birth has been completely validated in the scientific perspective of modern medicine. However, a number of these technologic methods and common practices have not been justified by scientific evidence. For some, not enough evidence has been obtained to prove that a particular method or practice is more helpful than harmful. For others, the accumulated evidence indicates that that method or practice can be actually injurious or dangerous.

Routine electronic fetal monitoring for labor: EFM began to be widely adopted around 1970, when it was viewed as a promising new technique for ascertaining fetal well-being in high-risk labors. Monitoring became more and more widely used in the following years, until it became routine for all labors in some hospitals—even though no scientific studies justified such use.

Eventually, a scientific analysis of the routine use of EFM was made by Albert Haverkamp, a physician specializing in obstretrics, and his colleagues. They reported their results in 1976 and 1977.[2] Dr. Haverkamp's study was designed to ascertain at just what point and under what conditions the electronic fetal monitor proved to be superior to humans using stethoscopes in labor.

Dr. Haverkamp and his associates were surprised by their findings. Use of the machine demonstrated no improvement in birth outcomes, a rate of birth by cesarean section three times that of human-monitored mothers, and a resultant increase in maternal and infant illness caused by the surgery. (The increase in surgical birth is especially alarming. The rate of maternal mortality runs on the order of 80 per 100,000 cases for c-section birth, compared to 27 per 100,000 cases for all women combined having either vaginal or c-section births. In other words, risk of mortality while small tends to almost triple in a cesarean.)[3]

When Haverkamp discussed his findings with colleagues, he was not honored but criticized. He commented in 1977:

> Five or six years ago, most obstetricians at scientific meetings were questioning the need for monitoring. Today, at the same meetings, if the efficiency and safety of monitoring are questioned, one is attacked as backward or ignorant. What was to be tested has, without clear evidence, become a basic assumption. This assumption is of concern not only because of the lack of scientific approach to a new strategy, but more importantly because of its implication for medical care.[4]

As an expectant parent, you cannot simply take it for granted that new technologic methods in pregnancy and birth are needed in your case or are risk-free. Try to avoid them unless a convincing argument for their necessity can be made.

Routine enemas and shaving of pubic hair: In the conventional birth procedures long used by many hospitals, workups for all women in early labor routinely include shaving of the pubic hair and administration of an enema, the purpose being to achieve the greatest possible cleanliness of the birth area and to reduce infection. Emptying the lower bowel is supposed to lessen risk of contamination from feces as the baby is born. But two recent studies in Great Britain indicate that neither practice realizes benefits.

In the study of shaving, 225 women were left to go through labor unshaved, 228 received a complete shave, and 240 were given a partial shave (of only the area immediately adjacent to the vaginal opening).

In reporting on the study, M. L. Romney stated that no significant difference was found in the frequency of infection among the three groups of women. In addition, 98 percent of the women shaved stated that the procedure had been disagreeable, embarrassing, or acutely uncomfortable. The author commented: "We find no evidence to support the current and widespread practice of perineal shaving. It increases patient discomfort without reducing infection or improving healing. We believe that perineal shaving is an unjustified assault and should be abandoned." [5]

A second study by M. L. Romney and associates investigated the routine administration of enemas to women in labor (A number of practitioners recommended the enemas not only to cut down on possible fecal contamination but also to stimulate uterine activity and descent of the fetus.)

This study involved 149 women who were given enemas and 125 who were not. Again, no significant differences resulted, including none in such key respects as frequency of infection or contamination and length of time in labor. Moreover, 84 women who had previously experienced childbirth were interviewed before the study, and all 84 said they preferred no enemas; 42 deemed the enemas "degrading and uncomfortable."

In their conclusions, the authors urged that the use of enemas be restricted to women in labor who "have an obviously loaded rectum palpable at the time of initial pelvic examination." They said that enemas given without valid medical reasons wasted time and resources while almost needlessly distressing some patients, and that in consequence "such rectal assaults on women in labor should be discouraged." [6]

The routine administrations of shaving and enemas clearly illustrate how distressing practices of conventional birth are not always clearly justified by scientific evidence.

Repeated cesarean deliveries: Since the early 1900s, obstetrical specialists have recommended that any woman who had had a cesarean birth absolutely must have any later deliveries also by cesarean section (c-section) in order to avoid rupture of the uterus during labor. (Such uterine rupture is fatal to the mother in about half of all cases in which it occurs.) The practice of repeat cesareans became virtually universal.

The incisions for c-sections in the early 1900s, and for many years after, were either the "classical" vertical one or the inverted-T incision, with combined vertical and horizontal cuts.

In recent years, however, a different type of incision, the low segment transverse incision, has been developed and has come into increasingly wide use. In the approach to the lower uterine segment, the incision through the skin runs horizontally at about the top of the pubic-hair line and has subtantial cosmetic as well as safety advantages. It is popularly termed "the bikini cut" since the scar it leaves usually cannot be seen even if the woman wears a bikini bathing suit.

But repeat cesareans still continued to be performed in more than 98 percent of all applicable cases.[7] In 1980, more than 175,000 of the 600,000 cesarean births in the U.S. were repeat cesareans.[8]

A few pioneering practitioners—with the cooperation and often the urging of expectant parents—saw distinct advantages to vaginal birth even after an earlier cesarean, however. They carried out studies and found that vaginal delivery could be successfully accomplished after a prior cesarean. One of their findings was that a bikini-cut scar on the uterus was less likely to rupture than were scars from the earlier types of incisions.

As a result of these studies—and of a conference held by the National Institutes of Health in 1981—the American College of Obstetricians and Gynecologists (ACOG) announced adoption of a significant new policy on repeat cesareans in 1982.[9] At the heart of the new policy was the position that "under proper conditions, many women who have had a cesarean birth may safely be considered for vaginal delivery." As a result of the new ACOG position, some 70,000 to 87,500 women a year who would very probably otherwise have had repeat cesareans may now have vaginal deliveries.

Just one beneficial result is a reduction in childbirth mortality. Repeat cesareans carry more than twice the risk of the mother's death in childbirth compared to the risk with vaginal birth.[10]

Announced with the new ACOG policy were official "Guidelines for Vaginal Delivery After a Cesarean Childbirth." [11] These include:

- documented low segment transverse incision (bikini cut) for the prior cesarean,
- nonrepeating reason for the prior cesarean,
- discussion early in pregnancy between the woman and her physician of options for a trial of labor, to allow for planning,
- expected birth of a single infant (rather than a multiple birth) and estimated birth weight of under 8.8 pounds,

- continuous electronic monitoring of fetal heartbeat and uterine contractions throughout labor, and
- understanding by the patient of the possible necessity of ending the trial of labor and switching to cesarean section.

The whole question of reducing the chances of having a cesarean birth—either an initial or a repeat cesarean—is treated extensively in a book by Christopher Norwood, *How to Avoid a Cesarean Section* (see Appendix B).

The Cultural Perspective

You may have been puzzled by our reports in the preceding pages. Why have practices in conventional hospital birth persisted when they are not justified by scientific evidence, you may wonder? Seeing those practices in a cultural perspective may give some answers to this and similar questions.

One fundamental point to understand is that each society or culture usually develops its own comprehensive way of carrying out its "rites of passage" such as weddings, coming of age, funerals, and also births.

Barbara Jordan, an anthropologist, has pointed out the internal consistency and compelling authority of the birth practices of any one culture:

> . . . It is not surprising . . . that—whatever the details of a given [culture's] birthing system—its practitioners will tend to see it as the best way, the right way, indeed *the* way to bring a child into the world. . . . We find that within any given system, birth practices appear packaged into a relatively uniform, systematic, standardized, ritualized, even morally required routine.[12]

As Dr. Lubic remarked in discussing "the American way of birth" in an earlier work: "Birth practices tend to become standardized around such aspects as accepted setting, attendants, and maternal position for parturition or 'birthing' to take place. Procedures or rituals regarding the immediate care of the newborn and the disposal of the placenta are found no less in the United States than elsewhere."[13]

This ethnocentricity is true also of American obstetrically oriented care—the conventional hospital alternative—which for the most part focuses on the potential for medical complications and on the management of the relatively few abnormalities.

When you understand the strength of this societal influence, you can see why the birth alternative you choose should appeal to you in a deep emotional way as well as intellectually. An alternative that appeals to you should be a good one for you—provided that you know what risks are entailed in your specific circumstances and you willingly accept those risks after considering them in the context of other available options. What helps make this suggestion reasonable is a broad conclusion based on experience and descriptive data:

> *Out-of-hospital birth alternatives today can carry risks no greater than (or even lower than) the risks would be with in-hospital alternatives, for the large majority of births that are normal or low-risk.*

Whatever choice you make, you will feel the impulse to find arguments and evidence in favor of it if its value or safety is challenged. And you'll feel compelled to find arguments against other alternatives that may be urged upon you. Health-care professionals are no different; many react the same way when their individual preferences are questioned.

Let us cite one example by way of illustration. In 1973 the Maternity Center Association began to investigate the desirability of introducing an out-of-hospital birth center as a demonstration project in response to the need for a birth alternative. Extremely thorough and sound plans and justifications for the proposed MCA center were made and then announced. Safety for prospective users was given particular attention. Based on MCA's twenty-eight years of experience in home birth (1931–1959), the safety factor was projected to be at least as high as it would be for comparable pregnant women having conventional hospital births.

The operation of the center was actively opposed by many physicians and obstetricians, through their professional organizations, particularly in New York. This opposition was carried out in spite of approval of the center by MCA's prestigious Medical Advisory Board.

A detailed analysis of the opposition was made by Dr. Lubic. She sought to show whether the opposition paralleled the patterns of action characteristic of any well established group, as reported in the findings of political anthropology. Carried out as her doctoral dissertation, the study documented many incidents evidencing clearly how the opposition reacted in a manner typical of any group faced with a real or imagined loss of control or standing.[14]

In other words, the study demonstrated that even professional scientists can be influenced more deeply by their cultural determined conception of the "right" way of birth than by their scientific judgment.

However, through more than ten years of operation and well over 2,000 births, the Childbearing Center has a safety record that is in fact at least as good as the records of leading hospitals with comparable pregnancies. We say "at least" for the reason that the opposition has prevented the comparative studies and trials necessary to make clear assessments. Because of the high level of controversy involved, a committee of the Institute of Medicine of the National Academy of Sciences reviewed the literature on the topic of birth settings and concluded that all settings need study.[15]

Why are various practices in conventional hospital birth, not justified by scientific evidence, still in wide use? Essentially, in our opinion, because of cultural biases within the medical subculture which views pregnancy as an illness to be aggressively managed.

Keys to Sound Conclusions on Birth Alternatives

As an expectant parent, how can you hope to reach sound conclusions on birth alternatives and practices for yourself, given your cultural bias? Just being aware of your bias helps you make allowances to offset it. Keeping an open mind protects you from automatically blocking out evidence or ideas that could prove valuable. Bias is also countered by staying as detached as possible while examining any body of evidence and the conclusions it logically implies.

While some cultural bias cannot be avoided, you can work to balance it by being alert to it. And such bias should not be entirely condemned. It's a primary source of the attachment, conviction, and enthusiasm with which we go about our preferred method of birth. Just try not to let it block consideration of other factors while you follow these steps in reaching your decision:

1. *Settle the basic question: Is this likely to be a low-risk, normal birth?* Only if it is, would it be advisable for you to consider out-of-hospital alternatives, such as home birth or freestanding birth centers.

   Certain conditions pertaining to the mother-to-be indicate the probability of something other than a low-risk, normal birth:

   • age 40 or older and due to have a first child, or 45 or older and expecting a second to fifth child

   • high blood pressure (chronic hypertension) or heart disease

   • diabetes mellitus

   • serious medical problems of some other kind

   • severe, recurrent migraine headaches

- current therapy for drug addiction
- substantially underweight or overweight.

If any of these conditions applies to you, you may be ineligible for enrollment at a birth center. Check with them for a specific evaluation.

2. *List your preferences in order:* Decide on the alternatives you prefer, and rank them according to your preference. List a preferred alternative even if you doubt if one of that type can be found in your locale. Searching could turn one up.

3. *Find out what varieties of birth alternatives, maternity-care professionals, and related prenatal classes are available in your vicinity.*

4. *Visit birth facilities and professionals representing alternatives that appeal to you:* Make appointments and actually visit the birth center, hospital, or office and talk with the personnel. On your visits ask for the names of parents who have recently used the service and would be willing to discuss their care. (You might also locate parents through acquaintances.) Your inquiries should be welcome. If they are not, you have learned something.

   For individual care-givers there may be no charge for a get-acquainted visit if you can be flexible in setting the time for an appointment.

5. *Go out of your way to make early arrangements for comprehensive prenatal classes:* Virtually all birth centers, many hospitals, and numerous other public-health agencies give prenatal classes for expectant parents. Find out what classes are available in your community.

6. *Taking all factors thoughtfully into account, make your choices:* After careful thought and discussion with those you trust, decide on your preferences for a specific birth setting, a care-giver, and prenatal classes. Try to get these choices settled no later than about your third month of pregnancy, earlier if possible. Checklists to help you choose are provided at the end of this chapter.

How to Find and Choose a Birth Setting

Be sure to look for offerings of any types of birth-setting alternatives that you think you might prefer. Don't assume that one or another kind may or may not be available until you make a systematic search. You should find your preferred type of facility or birth setting first, because the choices of care-givers and classes are often based on the type of facility chosen.

Finding an Out-of-Hospital Birth Center

To locate possible out-of-hospital birth centers in your vicinity, write to the National Association of Childbearing Centers (see Appendix A). Ask whether centers in your area are licensed and/or accredited. Most centers offer orientation sessions and provide brochures and other literature.

Finding a Hospital with Family-Centered Maternity Care

One approach for finding such hospitals is to ask one or more organizations dedicated to furthering family-centered childbirth, such as the International Childbirth Education Association (see Appendix A). As one of the services, the ICEA will provide information on family-centered maternity care in your area. When writing or phoning, you might ask for the address and phone number of its nearest local chapter (ICEA has some 300 chapters coast-to-coast). The professionals and parents who belong to a chapter in your locale should be able to advise you about specific hospitals and the features of family-centered care each may provide.

Other sources for information about area hospitals are the American Society for Psychoprophylaxis in Obstetrics and the American Academy of Husband-Coached Childbirth (see Appendix A).

Another source is the current edition of the *Registry of Nurse-Midwifery Services,* compiled and published by the American College of Nurse-Midwives. You might consult the book in a large public or college library nearby. (A copy may also be ordered from the ACNM at: 1522 K St. N.W., Suite 1120, Washington, DC 20005.) The hospitals with nurse-midwifery services listed there almost certainly offer maternity care that is at least somewhat family-centered in character. You could start with any hospitals it identifies in your locale and then ask those hospitals about specific features of their maternity-care provisions. Also, you could use the registry to locate nurse-midwifery services in your area, and then ask the person heading each service to suggest nearby hospitals that provide family-centered maternity care.

Finding a Hospital for Traditional Hospital Birth

To find hospitals offering conventional care, simply ask your family doctor or any physician specializing in obstetrics for the names of leading hospitals in your area that have maternity services. If you don't have a doctor, you can find an obstetrician in the Yellow Pages. When you are making inquiries, ask for the names of not only the hospital or hospitals where he or she is on staff, but of a few other leading or outstanding hospitals as well.

How to Find and Choose a Maternity Care-Giver

If you choose birth at home or at an out-of-hospital birth center, your choice will have a substantial influence on the professional care-giver you will engage. The feasibility of home birth might depend on whether you can find a suitable care-giver. If you choose a birth center, your major care-givers will be the professionals on the center's staff or affiliated with it.

Finding Care-Givers for Home Birth

Friends who have used a professional practitioner for home birth are your best source of information. As another possibility, you could seek professionals providing home-birth maternity care through organizations dedicated to home birth (see Appendix A). One group is the International Association of Parents and Professionals for Safe Alternatives in Childbirth. Among IAPSAC publications is the *Directory of Alternative Birth Services,* which lists names and addresses of physicians and midwives who provide prenatal and delivery care in home births. It also lists alternative birth centers and local IAPSAC chapters.

Always check information personally.

Finding Care-Givers for Birth at a Birth Center

If you settle on an out-of-hospital birth center as your birth alternative, you will probably receive most of your health care through pregnancy, labor, and birth from professionals affiliated with the center. Those providing the major part of your care will most likely be certified nurse-midwives working as full-time staff members. They will carry out an initial physical examination and will conduct periodic checkups every few weeks throughout the pregnancy.

Backing them up in this care will be one or more practitioners of obstetrics serving on the staff or as consultants. You will be able to consult with a center obstetrician as needed. (Birth centers operated by physicians are also being seen in greater numbers.)

For care of your baby after the birth, centers may require you to arrange for your own pediatrician (or other practitioner) six weeks before your expected birth date. Centers also often ask their expectant parents to make arrangements with a family physician should any health problems not related to the pregnancy arise.

Finding Care-Givers for Birth at a Hospital

It should be fairly simple for you to locate professionals providing maternity care for birth at a hospital—whether one with family-centered care or one with conventional maternity care.

You can take steps to find a care-giver while making an inspection visit to the hospital and talking to parents who have actually used it, as we have suggested. On your visit, ask experienced maternity nurses, as well as administrators in the maternity or obstetrical services office, to suggest staff physicians who meet certain criteria, for example:

- women physicians;
- physicians with

  professional fees within your range,

  long experience,

  unusual professional distinction in obstetrics,

  recent obstetrical training,

  a flexible outlook,

  a particularly strong attachment to those features of family-centered maternity care in which you are most interested.

Parents you talk to will probably know only about their own care-givers, but having their firsthand views about the quality of care they actually received can prove quite helpful.

Next, meet with a few of the most promising potential care-givers, and then draw on your judgment of their personal qualities plus all you have learned to make your choice.

The following checklist will help you select your maternity care-giver. You can make copies of it from the book, or copy the questions onto file cards that you can use for reference and note-taking. Asking for a description of usual patterns may eliminate the necessity to ask questions.

CHECKLIST FOR CHOOSING A MATERNITY CARE-GIVER
(See Index for page references to specific terms.)

General

1. Type of practice (check one):

   ☐ Individual; if so, whom can I reach when you're not available? _____

   ☐ Group; if so, who gives me care for what when? _____

2. For every medical procedure and medication you recommend, will you explain to my satisfaction the risks and benefits involved and allow me to accept or reject what you're recommending? _____

Prenatal Care

3. Will you permit and show me how to make basic checkups of my: ☐ weight; ☐ pulse rate; ☐ blood pressure; ☐ urinalysis; ☐ fetus and uterus size and position, by palpation?

4. Will you advise me on my:

   ☐ genetic history; how? _____

   ☐ obstetrical and sexual history; how? _____

   ☐ work and workplace, for pregnancy and health hazards; how? _____

   ☐ home and neighborhood, for pregnancy and health hazards; how? _____

   ☐ personal habits/activities/sports, for pregnancy and health hazards; how? _____

   ☐ preparation for labor and birth by exercises, reading, etc.; how?

   _____

   ☐ preparation and readiness for breastfeeding; how?

   _____

5. Do you recommend prenatal classes: ☐ for me; ☐ for my husband (or other support partner during labor and birth)? Notes: _____

   If so, what classes? _____

6. If my baby is breech, do you practice external version? Yes _____ No _____ Explain _____

7. Do you do vaginal breech births? Yes _____ No _____

   Under what circumstances? _____

Labor Care

8. Who will serve as my chief care-giver during labor and birth? __

   _____

9. Will I be allowed to stand, walk, squat, move around, and change position all through labor? _____

   If not, what positions will be allowed, and when? _____

10. Do you permit fluids and light nourishment by mouth during labor?

   _____

11. What will be my position for birth? _____

   _____

12. Do you routinely order electronic fetal monitoring of any kind during labor? _____

   Notes: _____

13. Will I be given pain-killers if I ask for them during labor? _____.
   What pain-killers would you use, and how would they be given to me? _____

   _____

14. Under what conditions would you recommend induction of labor, and why? _____

Birth Care

15. Will I be allowed to go through labor and birth in the same bed? _____. If not, what will I be shifted onto for giving birth?

   _____

16. Might forceps * or a vacuum extractor * be used in the birth? __

   Under what conditions do you think forceps or vacuum extractor would be necessary? _____

   _____

17. Is it likely that an episiotomy * can be avoided in my case? _____. How? _____

   If needed, what kind of episiotomy would probably be made? __

   _____

* See Chapter 13.

18. Will I be able to have all features of the Leboyer birth method, with: ☐ dim lights and quieted sounds in the birth room; ☐ breathing begun spontaneously by the baby; ☐ skin-to-skin contact between baby and parents right after birth; ☐ a warm-water bath for baby shortly after birth; ☐ time for bonding between baby and parents soon after birth?

19. Can I start breastfeeding right after birth? _____

20. Will the baby stay in the same room with me starting right after birth? _____

 If the baby should be taken away at times, what would the reasons be, and how often and how long would such times be? _____

21. Can we photograph the birth as it takes place? _____ Notes:
 _____

22. What is your opinion on circumcision? _____

23. If my baby has a problem, will I be able to touch and hold the infant? _____

24. What kind of eye prophylaxis is used? _____

25. Is vitamin K or any other medication routinely given to the baby?
 _____

Postnatal Care

26. How soon after the birth will we be allowed to go home? _____

27. Who will give me help with breastfeeding, if I need it? _____

 With preparation for bottlefeeding, if that's my choice? _____

28. What follow-up care will I get from you? _____
 _____

Fees and Payment

29. What is the fee for your care? _____

 Notes: _____

30. Can the fee be paid in installments, and if so, on what kind of schedule? _____
 _____

31. What kinds of health-care insurance coverage are acceptable for payment? _____
 _____

How to Find and Choose Prenatal Classes

Which kind of prenatal classes you select also depends to a substantial extent on the type of birth alternative you have chosen. For home birth, you can get information about classes for preparation from the organizations listed in Appendix A.

For birth at an out-of-hospital birth center, the center itself probably conducts classes that are required for persons planning to have their babies there. Some centers instead have their parents take classes elsewhere in prepared childbirth and parenting. Many centers have information on classes offered by other agencies in such techniques as special fitness, dance, or yoga exercises for pregnancy and birth.

If you've decided on a hospital birth, the hospital or the care-giver you've chosen may recommend a certain series of classes for you. You can also locate prenatal classes on your own by contacting one of the major organizations devoted to childbirth education (see Appendix A).

A checklist to help you choose prenatal classes is given on the following pages. Take along a copy of the checklist when visiting each class to see at first hand what it's like.

CHECKLIST FOR CHOOSING PRENATAL CLASSES

General

1. Which method of childbirth preparation is the one mainly taught in the classes? ☐ Lamaze; ☐ Bradley (husband-coached childbirth); ☐ Dick-Read (natural childbirth); ☐ combination of _____

   Notes: _____

2. Number of class sessions held (6 to 10 is desirable): _____

3. When do the class sessions meet (dates/days, starting time): _____

4. Length of each class session (2 hours is believed preferable—the first for lecture/discussion, the second for exercise coaching and practice): _____ Notes: _____

5. Participation in the classes by the husband (or other support partner) is: ☐ not permitted; ☐ permitted; ☐ recommended; ☐ required

   Notes: _____

133

6. Maximum enrollment for a class (about 10 couples is the advisable maximum): _____

7. Fee(s) charged for the classes (if any): _____

Teacher(s)

8. General professional background of the main (or only) teacher of the classes: ☐ Certified Nurse-Midwife; ☐ Registered Nurse; ☐ Certified Childbirth Educator; ☐ Other (specify) _____

   Name (if definite before you enroll) _____

9. Has the main (or only) teacher taken formal preparation as a childbirth educator from: ☐ ICEA (general); ☐ MCA (comprehensive); ☐ ASPO (Lamaze); ☐ AAHCC (Bradley)? Notes: _____

Content of the Classes

10. ☐ Explanation of the physical and emotional development of pregnancy, with wall-chart illustrations

11. ☐ Explanation of sound prenatal self-care and health care, including nutrition and use of drugs

12. ☐ Actions to take during pregnancy to promote comfort in pregnancy and relief of common complaints

13. ☐ Explanation of labor and birth in cases of normal, low-risk pregnancy, with wall-chart illustrations

14. ☐ Pros and cons of analgesia and anesthesia in labor

15. ☐ Explanation and practice of exercises to relieve pregnancy discomforts, to tone muscle systems for labor, and to rehearse exercises that will relieve pain and stress in labor and birth

16. ☐ All learning and practice of exercises, breathing methods, and relaxation techniques are performed together by the woman and her support partner

17. ☐ Explanation and practice of breathing methods for use by the woman with the help of her support partner during labor and birth

18. ☐ Explanation and practice of relaxation techniques for similar use during labor and birth

19. ☐ Explanation of possible complications in pregnancy and labor, and how to avoid them if possible, diagnose them, and cope with them

20. ☐ Explanation of cesarean birth and circumstances in which it would be necessary

21. ☐ Explanation of breastfeeding and preparing for it, and of bottle-feeding

22. ☐ Explanation of the rights of expectant couples in health care throughout pregnancy, labor, and birth, and of the choices open to them for this health care

23. ☐ Explanation of the care of the newborn in the minutes and days after the birth, including layette, bathing, feeding, jaundice, and circumcision

24. ☐ Couple and family interpersonal relationships

Specific Features of the Classes

25. ☐ Recommendation of basic books to read, and distribution to class members of supplementary study materials

26. ☐ Availability of many additional books and study materials at the facility where the classes are given

27. ☐ Showing of films of actual births of different types. Notes: _____

28. ☐ Inspection visits of actual birth facilities made: ☐ as recommended in class sessions; ☐ as part of a class session. Notes: _____

29. ☐ One or more couples from prior classes visit with their babies to discuss their birth experience. Notes: _____

30. ☐ Supplementary classes are ☐ required or ☐ strongly recommended. These are: ☐ La Leche League discussion group meetings (for breastfeeding); ☐ Lamaze breathing exercises classes; ☐ Other (specify): _____

31. ☐ Information about other classes of possible supplementary benefit or interest is provided (in such areas as dance exercises for pregnancy, other supplementary exercises, parenting, or nutrition). Notes: _____

32. ☐ To see how it all came out—and for the fun of it—is there a reunion of couples in the class with their new babies after they've all delivered?

II

Active Preparation for Birth

10

Prenatal Classes

Prenatal classes are essential, whether you're planning to have a family-centered birth with little or no anesthesia or any other form of delivery. In them you'll learn three kinds of skills: exercises to develop the fitness of your body in unique ways for pregnancy and birth, breathing and relaxation techniques that minimize pain during labor and birth, and teamwork methods for use by you and your husband (or other partner) that minimize pain during labor and birth and provide support in the postpartum period.

You will also learn a great deal that will contribute to an easier and more satisfying childbirth. Prenatal classes cover the major physical and emotional developments that you and your baby will be experiencing throughout pregnancy and birth. Knowing what to expect proves greatly reassuring and makes things manageable for most expectant mothers. You'll learn about the best ways to handle your common complaints and prenatal health care, and about preparation for and care of your baby. In really thorough classes, topics covered by most of the chapters of this book will be discussed. Classes then serve as a good reinforcement to your reading, and vice versa.

Prenatal classes also offer unique additional benefits from interaction with the teacher and with your classmates, the other expectant couples. Special questions that occur to you can be cleared up in talking with your teacher. Talking regularly with the other couples can give you many invaluable reactions and ideas. You're not likely to get such insights and inspiration on your own, and it's reassuring to know that others experience pregnancy as you do.

Besides, going through a prenatal class is a warmly human experience of a very rare kind. Friendships made in classes often prove particularly helpful to couples for mutual support in adjusting to early parenting.

Exercises for Fitness and Capability in Birth

Labor and birth will put you through vigorous physical exertion of rising intensity, rather like running a marathon with a final burst across the finish line. Of course you wouldn't dream of trying to run a marathon without first conditioning yourself for it. Similarly, you can learn in prenatal classes how to get in condition for the physical work of birth. You and your support person will learn how to collaborate on conditioning of four main kinds: prenatal exercises, relaxation methods, breathing techniques, and teamwork during labor and birth.

Your Prenatal Exercises—A Daily Program

In typical prenatal classes, you would be taught to do daily exercises along the line described here.* (Ask your prenatal health-care practitioner about these or any other special exercises before starting them, just to be safe.)

Carry out the exercise routine twice a day, every morning and every afternoon or night. In addition, do specific exercises any time you need them to relieve physical discomfort, as noted in the descriptions. Some of the exercises can be practiced at odd moments throughout the day, also as noted, for greater benefit.

Pelvic Rock: You can perform this exercise with your body in any of four positions—on all fours, as shown in Figure 10.1; when lying on your back; when sitting; or when standing erect. Practice it on all fours in your regular exercise routine, and use it in the other positions as needed to relieve discomfort.

Carry out these steps in slow, rhythmic motions:

1. Tighten your abdominal wall, pulling it in and up and tucking in your buttocks.

---

* Exercise instructions are adapted and illustrations are reproduced, with permission, from the booklet "Preparation for Childbearing," © 1985, Maternity Center Association.

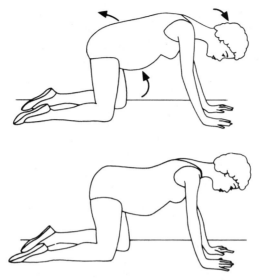

Figure 10.1.   Pelvic rock in the all-fours position

2. At the same time, rock the front of your pelvis upward toward your head so that your lower back arches outward.

3. Then, slowly relax your abdomen and buttocks, allowing your lower back to resume its normal, slight inward curve (but do *not* let your back curve sharply inward, and do *not* let your abdomen sag).

Do the pelvic rock exercise four to six times in your first sessions, and increase every third day by one more time until you're up to ten times per session.

This exercise helps relieve abdominal pressure and lower backache. You can use it from early pregnancy on into early labor. In later pregnancy, be especially careful not to let your back fall into a sharply swaybacked inward curve nor to let your heavy abdomen sag greatly.

Tailor-sitting and rib-cage lift: Take the tailor-sitting position (or modified yoga lotus position) as shown in Figure 10.2. Cross your legs, simply by folding one loosely inside the other. Or, even better, sit with the soles of your feet pressed together and your knees out as flat as possible to each side.

1. In a smooth, flowing motion, curve one arm up over your head as shown, and then bring it back to the starting position.

2. Do the same with your other arm.

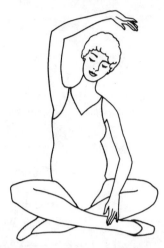

Figure 10.2. Tailor-sitting exercises: rib-cage lift

Do this rib-cage-lifting exercise eight to ten times in your first session, and increase by two every third day until you're up to fifteen times per session.

You get two kinds of benefits from this exercise. From tailor-sitting, you limber your upper leg joints and strengthen your thigh muscles. You should sit like this as often as possible during pregnancy instead of sitting in chairs—while reading, phoning, conversing, or watching TV, for example. Perhaps have a floor cushion or two handy to make it more comfortable.

From rib-cage-lifting, you benefit by relieving any pressure that develops under your ribs and by providing more breathing space as your uterus rises higher and higher in your abdominal cavity. The lifting also helps relieve tensed shoulder, neck, arm, or side muscles; use it any time you need to relieve such discomforts (particularly in standing or seated positions). In addition, regularly doing the lift exercise strengthens your shoulder and trunk muscles for later lifting and carrying your growing baby.

Tailor-sitting and leg-spread: Take the tailor-sitting position, but with the soles of your feet pressed together. Then:

1. Place your right hand under your right knee.
2. Pulling upward with your right arm, at the same time use your leg muscle to push your knee down toward the floor, against the pressure of your hand.

3. Hold your knee at its lowest point for a count of five.
4. Relax your leg and arm muscles and let your knee return to its original position.
5. Repeat the process with your left hand and leg.

Start with four or five pairs of leg-spreads per session, and every third day increase by one until you're doing ten per session.

In addition to the limbering effects of the tailor-sitting position, the leg-spread benefits you by strengthening the muscles of your thighs. This helps you to be able to widen your pelvic opening at birth.

"Kegels"—pelvic floor contractions: Do pelvic floor contractions (named Kegels for the physician, Dr. Arnold Kegel, who developed them a half-century ago to relieve urinary difficulties). Sit on a chair and carry out the exercise as follows:

1. Tighten the muscles around your anal opening as you would in holding back a bowel movement. Keep these muscles tight. Leave your buttock muscles relaxed.
2. Pull forward on the muscles around the vagina and at the same time make them squeeze in on the vagina, as you would in holding back urine. Leave your inner thigh muscles relaxed.
3. Hold both sets of muscles tight while counting to three, and then smoothly relax them.
4. Lift the entire pelvic floor by contracting the muscles starting from the back and continuing through the muscles to the front; hold the floor muscles taut while counting to three; and then let them smoothly relax.

Begin with four or five of these Kegels in your first sessions, and then increase by two every third day until you level out at ten per session.

Kegels directly tone some of the most important muscles you'll use in birth. Having them in good condition can greatly ease the baby's passage through the birth canal and might also enable you to avoid an episiotomy—the surgical incision to enlarge the vaginal opening often made to help the baby pass. Kegel exercises also help avoid serious complications caused by a very weak pelvic floor.

Practice Kegels at other times during the day—as many as thirty to fifty times a day, some authorities urge—while you're sitting, driving, standing at the sink, or lying down resting. It is especially good

143

to practice whenever you are urinating; once you've relieved the first heavy pressure, smoothly stop the flow and hold while counting to seven or up to ten, and then smoothly start the flow again.

Carry out another especially good practice during sexual intercourse by contracting your vagina around your partner's penis. As this suggests, the Kegel also represents one of the most important "sexercises" introduced in recent years.

There are other benefits to Kegels, beyond the ones you realize directly in birth and the enrichment of your sex life as suggested above. Continued Kegel exercises throughout your adult life can promote good health for your genital system after the birth and through the oncoming years. Authorities often recommend that all adult women should do twenty to fifty Kegels a day.

Perineal massage: Beginning at about the thirty-fourth week of pregnancy you and your partner may also want to use massage to prepare the tissues of the perineum for the stretching they will undergo at birth. Your care-giver can instruct you on this technique during an examination. Also there is an instructional booklet available from the International Childbirth Education Association (Appendix A).

Head and shoulders lift: Lie on your back with knees bent, arms down straight at your sides, and a pillow or cloth under your head (as in Figure 10.3), and then:

1. Tighten your abdominal muscles, and lift your head and shoulders as far as you comfortably can.
2. Hold your head and shoulders in place while counting to six and breathing naturally (do not hold your breath).
3. Let your shoulders and head fall back smoothly, and relax their muscles and all other muscles completely for a few seconds before the next lift.

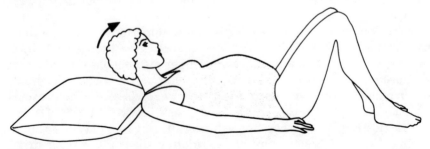

Figure 10.3. Head and shoulders lift

Do five lifts at your first session, and every three days increase by one up to ten lifts per session.

Head and shoulders lifts strengthen your abdominal muscles for their increasingly heavy load in pregnancy, without putting inadvisable strain on them.

You might be overstrained by doing sit-ups or leg-raises from a lying-down position in pregnancy. Don't try them unless you're expertly advised to do so.

Squat: From a standing position with your feet a short distance apart:

1. Lower your trunk smoothly down to a squatting position, with your weight on the balls of your feet, your knees held wide apart, and your buttocks almost or actually touching your heels (as in Figure 10.4). This is the same squat advised earlier for reaching things near the floor.
2. Remain squatting while you count to three and then rise smoothly to stand erect for a few seconds before your next squat.

Do five or six squats in your first session and then increase by one every third day until you're up to twelve per session.

Squatting practice limbers trunk and thigh muscles used in birth. The squat itself is also one of the most comfortable and healthful birth positions for the human body, and is commonly used in primitive cultures. You may find that you prefer a squatting position for birth.

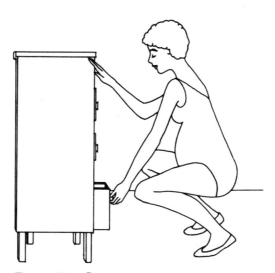

Figure 10.4. Squat

Using the squat during pregnancy instead of bending from the waist to pick up things at floor level also protects your back and abdominal muscles.

Shoulder circle: While sitting or standing, let your arms and hands hang loosely at your sides and:

1. Swing your shoulders together up toward your head (as in Figure 10.5).
2. Roll your shoulders back and down as far as they'll go without strain.
3. Let your shoulders move smoothly to their original position and again hang loosely relaxed for two or three seconds before doing the next shoulder circle.

Carry out four or five shoulder circles in your first session, and add one every three days until you're doing ten every session.

Regular shoulder-circle exercise strengthens your upper back and shoulder muscles and can help relieve upper backaches. It can also ease the numbness and tingling you may feel in your arms and hands from time to time, caused by the load pregnancy places on your circula-

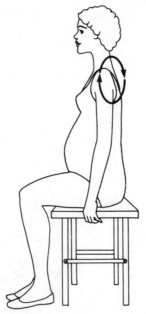

Figure 10.5. Shoulder circle

tory system. Use it whenever needed to help relieve upper backaches or numbness. Moreover, in late pregnancy this exercise can help relieve shortness of breath by providing somewhat more space for lung expansion.

Ankle circle: Sit in a chair with your legs propped up on a stool or another chair, and do as follows:

1. Let your feet hang beyond the edge of the stool, and rotate them at the ankles in the widest circles you can manage, first in a clockwise direction.
2. Pause, then rotate your feet in the opposite direction.

Rotate your feet about ten times in each direction per session.
Ankle circles improve circulation and relieve stiffness and swelling. Do them at any time you want to counter those conditions. If need be, you can do them while standing on each foot in turn (and holding on to something like a wall to keep your balance).

Prenatal Exercise Summary Checklist—Two Sessions Per Day

| | Times Per Session | | | |
	First Session	Every 3rd Day Increase by	Maximum	Do Extra as Needed for
Pelvic Rock	4–6	1	10	Abdominal pressure, lower backache
Rib-Cage Lift	8–10	2	15	Pressure under ribs, stiff neck, full breathing
Tailor Sitting	4–5	1	10	Comfort while sitting
Kegel	4–5	2	10	Pelvic muscle tone (do often)
Head and Shoulders Lift	5	1	10	
Squat	5–6	1	12	Picking up things from floor
Shoulder Circle	4–5	1	10	Upper backache, arm or hand numbness
Ankle Circle	10	—	—	Foot or ankle stiffness or swelling

Other Exercises

Many additional exercises are used in various kinds of prenatal exercise classes. If you're especially interested or active in dance, yoga, or physical conditioning, you may want to take a series of prenatal classes specializing in dance, yoga, aerobics, or conditioning exercise. What you learn could be built into your daily home exercise routines. It's wise to check out programs with your care-provider before you enroll.

Regular sports and active leisure pursuits such as swimming, walking, and dance can also provide valuable prenatal conditioning. You might want to spend even more time at these than usual, provided you don't strain, overexert, or run the risk of falling (and of course provided you have no physical condition making them inadvisable).

For aerobics or health-club exercise workouts, jogging, and yoga, you may continue if they were part of your pre-pregnancy regime, but listen to your body and be careful not to strain or overexert. With games you play regularly, such as golf or bowling, play in a relaxed rather than straining way. Games like tennis, badminton, and volleyball may be overstraining with a high risk of falling, as are softball and skiing.

Your Partner's Role in Prenatal Exercise

Your husband or other support person should carry out the role of comrade and teammate, learning basic exercises in class with you. At times, practice them together to improve understanding of the support role (not to mention his or her own conditioning). Your support person can encourage you to do your exercises regularly, and sometimes can do household chores to free your time for exercises.

Relaxation Methods for Pregnancy and Labor

Relaxation methods will probably be taught in your prenatal classes. Developing skill in these methods enables you to relieve the extra fatigue, strains, and muscular aches of pregnancy and to enjoy sound sleep. In labor, your relaxation skills can prove essential in managing and helping to eliminate pain.

Practice these relaxation exercises twice a day, either by yourself or with your partner. Use them to end your conditioning exercises in the morning if you like, or instead wait to do your morning set until around midday when you've grown tired and have developed some aches in your muscles. With your second daily relaxation exercises, either relieve late-afternoon fatigue and strain or do them in bed as a nightcap just before dropping off to sleep.

Whole-Body Relaxation

Methods or exercises for relaxing your entire body represent the first of two kinds of relaxation methods you can use by yourself. Both you and your partner should learn and practice these methods together, though, in order to make them fully effective. Carry out your exercise for whole-body relaxation in four stages, as follows.

1. *Lie down in a cushioned position:* Your body needs to be completely supported for you to become completely relaxed. In your first uses of whole-body relaxation, lie on your back or your side with your body cushioned, as shown earlier in Figure 7.8 and 7.9. After you develop this skill, you can also do it while sitting in a chair that supports your shoulders and head.

2. *Consciously relax each set of muscles from the top of your head to your toes:* Close your eyes or gaze at a fixed point, and at a leisurely pace start to relax each set of muscles, one by one, from the top of your head throughout your whole body—scalp, forehead, temples, eyebrows, eyes, ears, cheeks, mouth, jaw, tongue, neck front, neck rear, right shoulder, right upper arm, and so forth to the tips of your toes. Just let each set of muscles go limp.

   To tell if a certain set of muscles is relaxed, first tense that set tightly—tensing your forehead into a frown, for example, or your hand into a clenched fist. Then let those muscles relax more, and more, and more, until they're absolutely loose.

3. *Use basic relaxation breathing:* As you start to relax, take what we'll call a "complete" breath or "cleansing" breath. You take a complete breath in two steps: Inhale in a smooth, steady intake as deeply as you can. Then hiss or blow the air out as you exhale slowly, and at the same time let your whole body sink into relaxation.

   After your complete breath, go on with slow, quiet, rhythmic breaths of moderate depth.

4. *Control your state of mind:* Empty your mind of any worries, fears, annoyances, problems, reflections, enthusiasms, or excitement— any strong or changing feelings—while relaxing. Concentrate on something calm and constant, like a blank spot on the wall or the rhythm of your own breathing, with your eyes relaxed or lightly closed.

Remain relaxed for several minutes, or as long as you need to let your tiredness and aches ebb away. Continue your slow, rhythmic breathing.

When you are finished, take a second complete breath, a steady, deep one, and exhale slowly by hissing or blowing.

This breathing for whole-body relaxation is the type you should normally use through the start and early hours of your labor.

Selective Relaxation

Once you have mastered whole-body relaxation, you should start practicing a second kind of relaxation exercise that you can carry out by yourself. It develops skills you'll need specifically for labor.

Tense the muscles in one or two parts of your body while you relax the muscles in all the other parts of your body. For instance, go from whole-body relaxation to holding your entire right arm tense for several seconds while leaving all the rest of your body relaxed. Then relax your right arm completely, and leave the rest of your body relaxed while making your left leg muscles tense. Next, let those left leg muscles relax, tense both your right arm and your right leg, and keep the rest of your body relaxed.

After you can do this selective relaxation well, it is a good idea to carry out a daily exercise routine in which you successively tense and relax parts of your body as follows, all the time keeping the rest of your body relaxed:

1. right arm,
2. left arm,
3. right arm and right leg,
4. left arm and left leg,
5. right arm and left leg,
6. left arm and right leg,
7. both arms,
8. both legs.
9. Repeat the entire sequence three times.

Strengthening your ability to relax the parts of your body that are not being tensed helps you during labor. While your uterus tightens in each contraction, you use your newly developed ability to keep all of your other muscles relaxed.

Relaxation Exercises to Do with Your Partner

Whole-body relaxation: Your partner can help in two ways with your whole-body relaxation exercises. One is for him to do these exercises right alongside you, in order to learn at first hand how they feel and thereby become better able to guide you in using them. The second way is for him to serve as a quiet monitor, checking on how thoroughly you've relaxed. He would do this by touch, as in lifting your hand at the wrist a short distance and letting it fall limply, touching your shoulder or cheek to see if it's relaxed, or turning your foot a little from side to side with his hand. His touching and gentle moving of parts of your body should deepen your relaxation, rather than distract you from it.

He should also quietly say soothing, peaceful things to you; hushed, calm talk will prove especially effective in helping relaxation.

Partial-body relaxation: Your partner can also join in on the exercises in which you practice holding one or more parts of your body tense while relaxing all the rest of your body. In this, he or she touches one or two parts of your body—such as your left arm or right arm or left leg, and says to tense those body parts—and then, after you've tensed them for two or three seconds, he touches them again and says to relax completely. Your partner next goes on to have you tense other parts of your body, perhaps doing so in the order of a daily exercise routine you've developed.

Touch relaxation: A further development of this joint partial relaxation method, called "touch relaxation," is taught in a number of prenatal classes. You might find it unusually powerful for helping to relieve tension and pains during pregnancy and labor.

In it, your partner presses firmly on a part of your body that aches or is tense—for instance, on your shoulders at the end of a tiring day or at the sides of your head if you have a tension headache. Little by little, he gradually decreases the pressure while telling you quietly that your tension and pain are flowing out of you through his hands and away. Stroking movements down the full length of your arm or your inner thighs can similarly be used to ease tension in your upper arms or legs.

Practicing partial relaxation and touch relaxation with your partner develops skills that often prove particularly important in labor. With them, your partner can watch for parts of your body in which unnecessary strains are building up—perhaps your neck and shoulders, or your lower back or buttocks—while you're absorbed in the contractions and effort of labor. By touch and talk practiced together in relaxation exercises, your partner can help bring very welcome relaxation and relief back into those parts of your body. In the weeks of practicing touch relaxation before labor, be sure to work out with your partner exactly how much pressure and what kinds of touching and stroking best relieve tension and relax each part of your body. Touch relaxation is a technique that was developed in large part by a well-known British childbirth educator and author, Sheila Kitzinger.

Effleurage: A technique in which either you or your partner lightly massages your abdomen during labor is often taught in prenatal classes, especially in those using the Lamaze approach. It helps ease abdominal tension during contractions in labor, and can also be comforting for such tension in the later months of your pregnancy.

1. Massage gently by moving the fingertips in steady, light circular motions starting below your navel or just above your pubis. It's best done on your bare skin, using a powder (cornstarch or talcum) to reduce friction and massaging with one or both hands.
2. Slowly move the hands outward along your groin, then upward to your rib cage, inward along the bottom of your ribs, and down the center to the starting point.
3. Repeat massaging along this overall pattern for several minutes at a time during pregnancy, or through a contraction in labor.

In labor, effleurage can help keep you from feeling discomfort from the power of labor contractions deep inside.

Reverse roles: In doing relaxation exercises with your partner, exchange roles from time to time. This will help each of you to understand the other's role and thereby better carry out your own.

Breathing Techniques for Labor and Birth

Most couples who successfully go through low-risk, prepared childbirth without anesthetics today find that they can do so largely because of the breathing techniques they learned in prenatal classes. You can master these special ways of breathing for labor by practicing them for about half an hour a day during pregnancy. Carry out as much of this practice as possible with your partner. And start the practice as early as possible after mid-pregnancy.

These techniques are tools for you to individualize for your own use. They may help when applied exactly as presented here. However, feel free to experiment with what helps you most at any given time. You need not be doctrinaire about it. You may well work out your own pattern of breathing techniques in the first-stage labor. Staying relaxed and in control of your breathing is more important than breathing in some specific way at a specific time.

In addition, in labor itself another partner will be helping on your support team—your professional care-giver, whom you have carefully chosen for his or her commitment to meeting your requests. The care-giver, working along with you and your personal support partner, reports on physical developments so that you can connect the facts of cervical effacement and dilation, and of descent of the baby through the pelvis, to what you are feeling and doing. In this section we emphasize the latter—what you should be doing. Your care-giver will help you apply and adapt these skills when labor comes.

Breathing for First-Stage Labor

The first type of breathing will give you the confidence and strength to handle the initial contractions of your uterus after labor begins. Those contractions will start almost unnoticeably, but will get more intense, longer, and more frequent as the hours pass. In normal childbirth, labor begins all by itself any time between two or three weeks before and two after the due date.

How to tell if you're in first-stage labor: You should generally be able to tell if labor has begun by these signs (although what causes labor to start remains incompletely known to science):

- *Vaginal discharge, or "show":* a discharge from your vagina of perhaps a quarter-cupful of mucus that is clear except for red tinges or streaks of blood. Called "show," this discharge represents the release of a mucus plug that has sealed your cervix during pregnancy. Contractions of the uterus start to stretch, or dilate, your cervix for birth, breaking loose the mucus plug. (For some women, the mucus plug is loosened but the show is not discharged for a number of days; for others, the mucus plug does not pass until they're so far advanced in labor that they hardly even notice it.)

- *Uterine contractions:* contractions of your uterus that go on for a number of hours and keep getting steadily stronger, longer, and more frequent. Such continued contractions are the surest sign of labor.

You or your partner should check the contractions with a watch or clock. Time how many minutes elapse between contractions and how many seconds each contraction lasts from start to finish.

You may find at the outset that contractions come 10 minutes, 8 minutes, or even only 5 minutes apart, and last some 30 seconds from the time they start gripping your uterus until it relaxes again. These contractions may feel like recurring backache, gas pains, or digestive cramps. Check to see if the uterus is contracting by putting your hand on your abdomen when you have the sensation.

Contractions that last about 40 or 50 seconds usually indicate that labor has begun in earnest. These contractions may come just 5 or 3 minutes part.

You may have experienced contractions somewhat like these with the series of lighter and passing Braxton-Hicks contractions that you can experience at intervals in the later months of pregnancy. Such "rehearsal" contractions fade to a stop after a few minutes (or hours), but may be sufficiently strong and long to lead you to think that labor has begun.

- *Rupture of the membranes: breaking of the amniotic sac, or "bag of waters," with the water flowing out (up to a few cupfuls, but it may seem like more). This may come as a gush or a trickle. It may also happen a number of days before labor actually starts, or after labor contractions are well along and you're in the birth center, hospital, or home birth-bed. Be sure to tell your care-giver as soon as it happens or you think it may have.*

Exercises for first-stage breathing: You already know the kind of breathing to use during contractions in early first-stage labor—it's much the same as the "basic relaxation breathing" that you use for your whole-body relaxation. (Figure 10.6).

1. *Start and end with a deep "cleansing breath."* Use a deep "cleansing breath" or "complete breath" to begin and to close. This is a breath for which you inhale as deeply as you can and then smoothly exhale while hissing or blowing.

2. *Take slow, deep breaths in between:* After the deep cleansing breath to start, go on by taking deep, slow, rhythmic breaths, and finally close with another especially deep cleansing breath.

For the full exercise, use this deep breathing over time spans like those of actual contractions you'll have in labor. Base your practice first on contractions running 30 seconds long, and later on contractions running 40 seconds and then 50 seconds long. Use a tailor-sitting position for the exercise, or one in which you're lying down but half propped up by pillows and with your legs stretched out straight or bent up at the knees and slightly apart. After repeating steps 1 and 2, completely relax for about a minute, and then repeat the breathing exercise through the time of another contraction. Repeat three to five times during each of your daily exercise sessions.

When you're practicing this and other breathing exercises for labor, your partner can use the following method to simulate the sensation of actual contractions. You could also do this when you're exercising alone.

To indicate the start of a contraction, your partner takes hold of a fairly thick pinch of flesh on the inside of your thigh between thumb and forefinger and at the same time quietly says, "Contraction starts." He or she goes on to indicate the time elapsed: "fifteen seconds . . . thirty seconds . . ." and finally, "contraction ends." At the same time he or she gradually presses harder to indicate how the contraction builds, and then eases off on the pressure to suggest its waning.

The next breathing exercise, which is for managing more active labor, follows the pattern depicted in Figure 10.7.

1. *Start with first-stage breathing:* At first use your first-stage type of breathing (slow deep breathing) through a first contraction time

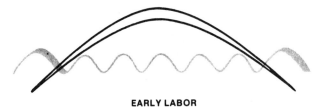

EARLY LABOR

Figure 10.6. Basic relaxation breathing

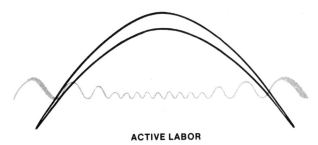

ACTIVE LABOR

Figure 10.7. Modified breathing for active labor

of 50 seconds. (In actual labor, you may continue with this deep breathing as long as it feels comfortable; some women find it effective all through labor.) After the 50-second contraction time, do whole-body relaxation and normal breathing for 30 seconds.

2. *Shift to light, high-chest breathing:* For a second contraction time of 60 seconds, assume that you're having a stronger contraction and do as follows:

As the contraction starts, take a deep cleansing breath, and hiss or blow to let it out slowly while relaxing completely. Then with each of the next several breaths, make it less and less deep until you're breathing mainly high up in your chest. This light, shallow breathing is sideways breathing, in a sense, for it moves your ribs in and out sideways while your abdomen stays still. (Your or your partner can verify the sideways movement by holding hands on your ribs and abdomen while you're doing it.)

Use a speed for this light breathing or chest breathing that's comfortable for you. If the breathing makes you dizzy or lightheaded, breathe more slowly and evenly, for you're getting too much oxygen (called hyperventilating). If it gives you too little air or you have trouble keeping it up in a regular rhythm, take one quick deep breath and then continue the light breathing.

Continue this light breathing through most of the 60-second contraction time, and as the contraction subsides while nearing its end, make each of four or five breaths successively deeper.

3. *End with a deep cleansing breath:* End these increasingly deep concluding breaths after the 60-second contraction time with a deep cleansing breath (one inhaled smoothly and exhaled slowly with hissing or blowing) while you go limp with whole-body relaxation. (Such opening and closing deep breaths are important for helping give the baby a large enough oxygen supply.)

4. *Repeat for 75-second contraction times:* Carry out whole-body relaxation for 60 seconds, and then repeat this light breathing through a next contraction time of 75 seconds. Again use whole-body relaxation for 60 seconds, and repeat this breathing for another 75-second contraction.

Breathing for Transition

How to tell if you're approaching transition: Through first-stage labor your cervix gradually dilates, or stretches open, around the baby's head to allow the baby to pass through in birth. Successive contractions of the uterus little by little dilate the cervix until it is 10 centimeters in diameter—about 4 inches—large enough to let the baby's head through.

First-stage labor is the time span over which your cervix dilates to that full opening of 10 centimeters. Near the end of first-stage comes a shorter but often difficult span called transition. Transition gives way to second-stage labor, in which you deliver your baby.

You can tell if you're nearing and entering transition by these signs:

• *Contractions of 1 minute or more coming close together:* Contractions intensify to some 50 and 60 seconds long with shorter (3-minute) intervals between as your cervix dilates to 6 to 8 centimeters while approaching transition. As your cervix dilates up to 10 centimeters during transition, the contractions continue to grow stronger, longer, and closer together. They run 60 to 75 seconds long and may come only 30 seconds apart in transition itself.

• *Feeling of panic and being under great stress:* Guidance on breathing and comforting actions by your partner prove important in relieving the sense of panic and of being under heavy stress that you will probably feel during transition.

The very heavy, strong contractions may make you irritated, hot, sensitive to annoyances, and confused. You may have uncontrollable tremors in your legs, or a feeling of nausea. You may also feel an urge to push as the baby descends and puts pressure on your rectum. But it is important not to push until the cervix is fully open.

Concentration on breathing, on your partner's coaching instructions, and on getting through one contraction at a time—all these will help lead you to the usually easier time of second-stage labor and birth.

Transition breathing: For transition breathing, follow the active labor pattern in Figure 10.7 on page 155, but when you do the light high-chest breathing, puff out as you exhale on every third or fourth breath.

Breathing for Second-Stage Labor

How to tell if you're in second-stage labor: Two main signs will probably mark your shift from transition into second-stage labor:

• *Relief:* A sense of relief and confidence should replace the feelings of confusion and stress you had during transition.

• *Strong urge to push as part of your contractions:* Your contractions will continue to be strong but may well come at longer intervals, so you will have more time to rest between them. With them you will probably start feeling a powerful urge to push down with your system and expel the baby. (However, some women do not have such feelings.)

Not pushing when told not to by your professional partner, and pushing as much as possible when you're told to push, will be important actions for you to take. Your second-stage breathing techniques play an essential part in your ability to not push and to push.

Exercises for second-stage breathing: First, practice "panting breathing" (Figure 10.8) for second-stage labor, as follows:

1. Assume a 70-second contraction time, and start by taking two cleansing breaths.
2. Take a deep breath, and keep your jaw, shoulders, legs, and pelvic floor relaxed.
3. Breathe in and out very quickly with your mouth open, like a panting dog.
4. Continue breathing in this fashion for a brief period.
5. Relax and repeat steps 2, 3, and 4 as many times as you need until the contraction ends.
6. Take two cleansing breaths as the contraction ends, and then rest in whole-body relaxation.

Those steps 2, 3, and 4 can effectively counter your urge to push by keeping the diaphragm high. It's impossible to push while panting. Second, practice "pushing breathing" for second-stage labor:

1. Assume a 70-second contraction, and start by taking a cleansing breath; then take a second cleansing breath (which you would take in actual labor only if you are able to before the contraction grips you).

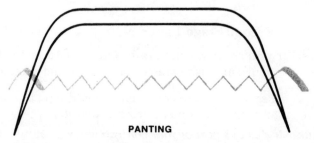

PANTING

Figure 10.8. Panting breathing

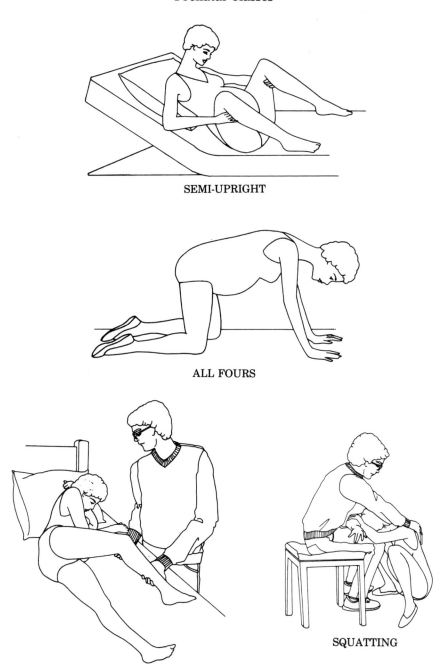

SEMI-UPRIGHT

ALL FOURS

SQUATTING

SIDE-LYING

Figure 10.9. Positions for pushing in second-stage labor

2. Take a deep breath, scooping it in, and hold it.

3. Quickly drop your chin, round your shoulders, pull in your abdominal muscles, rock your pelvis up, and stick your elbows out to the sides while pulling your legs up and apart with your hands. This position can be taken while you're sitting up or squatting.

4. For the exercise, hold the position while continuing to hold your breath for 5 or 6 seconds. Do *not* bear down during your pregnancy. (However, in labor, you would tighten your abdominal muscles and push the baby toward your relaxed pelvic floor muscles.)

5. After the 5 or 6 seconds, release the remaining air with a grunt while pulling your abdominal muscles in more tightly.

6. Raise your head, scoop in another quick deep breath, and hold it for 5 or 6 seconds.

7. Repeat the process in steps 4, 5, and 6 until the urge to push is gone and the contraction is over.

8. Take two cleansing breaths when the contraction is over.

Breathing through Birth and Third-Stage Labor

You won't need any additional breathing techniques to help you through your baby's birth at the end of second-stage labor, nor through third-stage labor, in which the placenta is expelled and the uterus rises in your abdomen. Through these culminating phases of labor, your care-giver will ask you to use the kinds of breathing you've already mastered—mainly the not-pushing, pushing, or whole-body relaxation varieties.

Teamwork through Labor and Birth

In prenatal classes, you and your partner will learn still more ways to develop and improve your teamwork through labor and birth. You'll see what these are in Chapter 13, "Labor and Delivery and Giving Birth." And be sure to develop your teamwork skills by regularly joining each other in doing the exercises for conditioning, relaxation, and breathing as explained in this chapter.

11

Getting Ready to Feed
Your Baby

You and your partner will also prepare for feeding your new baby in comprehensive prenatal classes. You'll start by deciding between breastfeeding and bottlefeeding (or some combination of the two, as your situation may require).

Should You Breastfeed?

While it cannot be said that modern science discovered breastfeeding, it certainly has been successful in analyzing its many advantages.

Over the decade of the 1970s, breastfeeding more than doubled in popularity, as documented in population surveys by the U.S. Centers for Disease Control. Findings showed that in 1980, 51 percent of white mothers fed their babies entirely at breast as compared to only 19 percent in 1969. Corresponding figures for black mothers showed 25 percent breastfeeding exclusively in 1980 compared to only 9 percent in 1969.

The more highly educated the parents, the larger the proportion who chose breastfeeding, according to the surveys. Of women with only high-school education, between 17 and 44 percent were breastfeeding in 1980; for women with graduate-school education, the range was between 50 and 68 percent.[1]

Reasons for Breastfeeding

Benefits to infants: Features of breastfeeding that have persuaded increasing numbers of parents to favor it over bottlefeeding include these advantages:

- *Immunities to diseases:* Breastfeeding transmits the mother's immunities to the baby through her colostrum, a creamy, yellow precursor to true milk that is the first nourishment available to the baby. (You may first see colostrum as a sticky liquid on your nipples in your last weeks of pregnancy. A few days after you have your baby, it will be followed by your milk. How soon depends on how much suckling the baby is permitted.)

  Supplies of antibodies that protect against both viruses and bacteria continue to flow to the baby with the breast milk. Moreover, should the infant catch an infectious disease from a source other than the mother, and the organisms pass to her during nursing, the mother's system will generate antibodies in her milk to fight off the disease.

- *Helps protect against allergies:* In addition, breast milk helps protect the baby from allergic skin rashes, asthma, and allergic reactions to food, particularly to the protein found in breast milk substitutes. Parents who themselves suffer from allergies may want to give serious consideration to choosing breast milk and avoiding more highly allergenic cow's milk proteins.

- *Reduces chances of colic, vomiting, diarrhea, colds:* Babies fed at breast develop such infant ailments as colic, vomiting, diarrhea, ear infections, and upper respiratory infections less often than do bottlefed babies.

- *Ideal nutrition:* The mother's milk is automatically compounded in her system to provide just the right amounts and proportions of almost all the nutrients the baby needs—on two conditions: (1) she follows a reasonably sound diet for nursing mothers (taking some supplementary vitamins and minerals may be advisable, depending on her circumstances and diet), and (2) she avoids ingesting harmful medications or other substances whenever possible; such substances go directly into the baby's system with the milk, in some cases at proportionately much higher concentrations than in the mother's system.

  Babies do not become allergic to their mothers' milk (although some may develop severe allergies to cow's milk).

162

- *Fosters good dental and facial growth:* As a physical exercise, the infant's sucking on the breast may help to promote the correct alignment of dental arches and palates, as well as proper development of the facial structure.

Benefits to mothers: For mothers, breastfeeding has advantages over bottlefeeding that include:

- *Effect on the mother's figure:* Some women think breastfeeding will result in a less attractive figure, with sagging breasts and extra body fat. This is untrue.

While breasts are more full during pregnancy and breastfeeding, they will not lose their tone if women wear bras with certain features: (1) a cup size about one size larger than usually worn before pregnancy, and a fit around the ribs that is not too tight (the rib cage measurement usually expands in pregnancy, and often stays slightly larger in diameter after birth); (2) wide shoulder straps that don't constrict; (3) adequate under-breast support; and (4) a flap or panel with a catch that you can open and close easily with one hand. (If a nursing bra has a plastic liner, either take out or use another bra because the plastic cuts off air circulation and may lead to sore nipples.) If you find it necessary because of colostrum production, you can start to wear nursing pads (or pads of soft, absorbent cloth) over your nipples inside your bra during pregnancy.

As for body fat, breastfeeding rids you of your few pounds of extra pregnancy fat rather quickly.

Smaller-breasted women may welcome having larger breasts in pregnancy, but they also may assume that they can't produce enough milk for their babies. That is not correct. Breast size depends on the amount of fatty tissue rather than the number of milk-secreting glands. In fact, such women usually can breastfeed quite successfully.

- *Less bleeding, faster uterine recovery, after birth:* Breastfeeding your baby right after birth triggers the release of the hormone oxytocin into your system, causing the uterus to contract faster and reducing chances of hemorrhage. It also shortens the fifteen- to twenty-day postpartum vaginal discharge called lochia. Continued nursing helps your uterus to involute, or shrink, to the size it had been before pregnancy faster than if you were not breastfeeding.

- *Some, but not certain, contraceptive effect:* Women who breastfeed totally (giving no supplementary nursing bottles nor solid foods) rarely become pregnant until after they have their first menstrual period some six months postpartum.

However, you cannot be certain that breastfeeding will prevent conception. For contraception, use a condom with vaginal spermicidal foam or jelly, a newly fitted diaphragm, or the rhythm method as advised by a health care provider if you and your partner want to avoid getting pregnant. In general, birth-control pills should not be used because they can affect your milk production and their components also pass to the baby. Some care-providers consider the "mini pill" safe after feeding is well-established; get advice before making a decision. Because you won't be having regular periods, the rhythm method should be practiced based on examination of cervical mucus. Your care-provider should be able to instruct you.

- *Convenient and inexpensive:* Milk directly from the breast is always ready and always just right for the baby. It need not be bought, mixed, stored, warmed, or checked for possible spoilage. And the only cost is the extra food (and perhaps vitamin supplements) you consume in order to ensure good nutrition while nursing.

- *Deep personal satisfaction:* Women who freely choose to breastfeed usually derive much personal satisfaction from knowing that they are providing their baby with the best nutrition possible. They find a sense of fulfillment in following the natural, healthful sequence of pregnancy, birth, and nursing and in satisfying the baby's needs in a comforting and relaxing way.

Pediatricians officially recommend breastfeeding: Breastfeeding has been proven to have so many benefits that the professional organizations of pediatricians in the U.S. and Canada have jointly endorsed its use. In a statement issued in 1979 by the American Academy of Pediatrics (AAP) and the Canadian Paediatric Society (CPS), it was stated that the two groups "strongly recommend breastfeeding. . . . We believe human milk is nutritionally superior to formula. . . . The overall nutritional superiority of human milk remains unchallenged." Their statement further recommended breast milk for its powers to safeguard infants against illness.

On the emotional values of breast feeding, the joint statement declared: "Early and prolonged contact between a mother and her newborn infant can be an important factor in mother-infant bonding and the development of a mother's subsequent behavior to her infant."

Reasons Against Breastfeeding

Expectant parents may have some reasons for deciding against breastfeeding:

- *Too much trouble when the mother must work:* An urgent need, often financial, for the mother to resume work outside the home as soon as possible after having the baby can discourage breastfeeding for a number of couples.

- *Opposition of husband or other family members:* Breastfeeding requires the cooperation of your partner. Attitudes of other family members can also be discouraging, and should be fully discussed with them before arriving at your decision.

- *Mother's medicinal regime:* In cases where the mother has a chronic health condition requiring regular medication, breastfeeding is inadvisable if her medicines are among the many kinds harmful to nursing infants, such as antibiotics (Streptomycin, Chloromycetin, sulfadiazine and other sulfonamides, tetracyclines including Achromycin, Aureomycin, and Terramycin); nasal or bronchial decongestants (many types are either insufficiently investigated or disapproved for nursing mothers); and tranquilizers, antidepressants, and other drugs used in psychiatry.

  If you need to take medicines, do not rely on any published list like this, however, for guidance on what may be hazardous to your baby when nursing. Ongoing research is constantly developing important new findings. In order to learn of any recent developments that might apply in your case, ask your physician or other health-care provider about the safety of the specific medicines being proposed for you. Authoritative answers to questions about hazards may also be obtained by writing to the Professional Advisory Board of La Leche League International (see Appendix A).

- *Environmental pollutants in the mother's milk:* In some parts of the country, the breast milk of nursing mothers has been found to contain concentrations of environmental pollutants that are above levels defined as harmful. Among these are such pesticide residues and toxic industrial chemicals as DDT and PCBs. Expectant mothers in areas where large quantities of hazardous pollutants like these have been discovered may well have good reason not to breastfeed.

- *Feelings of modesty:* Concern about the possible necessity of exposing your breast to feed the baby in public (or even among friends of the opposite sex) may influence your decision.

- *Too confining for the mother:* Some expectant mothers think they would be too tied down by the need to breastfeed their babies as often as every two to four hours, day and night, perhaps for several weeks in the early days when most new mothers would be at home in any event. It is unquestionably confining.

165

Answering the Objections

You need not accept these arguments against breastfeeding as final if you want to nurse. Here are ways in which other women have gotten around these objections.

- *Countering "Too much trouble when mother must work"*: Increasing numbers of women find it practical to hold full-time jobs and still continue breastfeeding their babies. They usually take advantage of a maternity leave granted by their employers and spend at least several months at home. They then have a loving, familiar person care for the baby while mother works. (Such a person may not be easy to find and should be sought during pregnancy.)

  For feedings while she's at work, the mother may express milk from her breasts by hand or with a breast pump the day before. She can do this at work in a ladies' lounge. As soon as her milk is drawn, she bottles and refrigerates it. At the day's end she carries the bottles home, where it's kept refrigerated until the baby needs it, but not longer than 24 hours.

- *Countering "Opposition of husband or other family members"*: One of the most effective ways to disarm your husband's objections to breastfeeding is to have him attend prenatal classes with you. Learning from classmates, the teacher, your care-giver, and from reading about the marked values of breastfeeding can influence him to change his mind. Those who operate prenatal classes should welcome your family members.

- *Countering "Mother's medicinal regime"*: Mothers can generally solve this difficulty by asking their professional care-giver for advice regarding the timing of doses or about substitute drugs that can be used with safety.

- *Countering "Environmental pollutants in the mother's milk"*: The La Leche League International urges that you do not overreact to possible pollutant hazards in breast milk. No evidence of harm to breastfed babies from such causes has been conclusively reported, as far as we know.

  In testimony at U.S. Senate hearings on environmental toxins and breastfeeding in 1977, La Leche reports, the American Academy of Pediatrics stated: "There are no known effects in children at levels found in people in the United States."

However, the League recommends taking these steps in order to minimize your exposure to pollutants:

1. In your home, stop using insect poisons and other chemical sprays; laundry soaps, bleaches, softeners, and other laundry substances containing chemicals; and chemicals used to treat clothes to resist moths and wrinkling, and to waterproof clothes.

2. Do not wear permanently mothproofed clothes (which may contain dieldrin, a harmful substance).

3. Wash fruits and vegetables thoroughly under running water to remove pesticide residues (or peel them, although doing so removes vitamins).

4. When pregnant and breastfeeding, do not eat freshwater fish from waters known to be polluted; cut the fat off any meat you eat, because any toxic pollutants it may contain would be concentrated largely in the fat; and do not start on a drastic diet to reduce your weight quickly, because rapidly decomposing fat could release relatively large amounts of the pollutants stored in your fat, which could be picked up to some extent in your breast milk. It is also wise to contact your state or local health department if you have any concerns.

- *Countering "Feelings of modesty"*: It is simple to breastfeed a baby in public without exposing your breast. A coat, jacket, cloak, or scarf can cover your chest and the baby while you sit. Garments can be worn that easily unsnap or unzip for feedings, or sweaters can be pulled up.

- *Countering "Too confining for the mother"*: If you want to free yourself to go out for an evening or for a morning or afternoon, you can (as stated before) express some breast milk into bottles and keep it refrigerated. Accustom your baby to the bottles and to the baby-sitter gradually.

    A second possibility would be to introduce the baby to a nursing bottle filled with formula rather than breast milk. Doing so would not be as desirable for nutrition and health as using breast milk in bottles; the baby also might prefer breast milk.

    Another alternative is to take the baby along with you. You will find that it's easy to take small babies many places, including family or neighborhood restaurants.

167

Should You Bottlefeed?

Reasons for Bottlefeeding

These features of bottlefeeding might interest you:

- *Adequate nutrition if the mother cannot breastfeed:* If due to illness or emergency the baby's mother cannot nurse, bottlefeeding will of course provide adequate nutrition for health and growth.
- *Less confining for the mother:* Mothers who bottlefeed can lead less confining lives because they can go out and have their babies fed when hungry by baby-sitters.
- *Sharing in the satisfaction of feeding:* Daddy, grandparents, older brothers and sisters, and other relatives and friends can share in the satisfaction of feeding a new baby who's used to bottlefeeding.
- *More uninterrupted sleep for the mother:* Dad can also help Mom get more unbroken sleep through the night by taking some of those night feedings.
- *Measured amounts:* Bottlefeeding enables mothers to record with ease exactly how many ounces of formula the baby has taken at each feeding, just by looking at the ounce marks on the bottle. With breastfeeding you can tell if your baby has had enough only by the way he or she reacts.
- *Possible faster growth:* Some authorities claim that bottlefed babies grow faster and gain more weight than breastfed babies over the same time span. A related claim is that bottlefed babies can eat more at each feeding and can hence go longer between feedings. These claims have not been documented authoritatively as yet, however.

Reasons against Bottlefeeding

On the other hand, there are some less desirable aspects to bottlefeeding your baby. As explained in the discussion on breastfeeding, bottlefed babies miss the nutritional and immunological advantages of breast milk. Bottlefed babies are also more vulnerable to feeding ailments and allergies.

- *Celiac disease:* A history of celiac disease (an inherited malady marked by lagging development in the baby's digestive system) in the family of either parent usually leads health-care-givers to advise breastfeeding.

- *Risk of overfeeding:* Concern about making sure the baby gets enough to eat may lead mothers to use bottlefeeding and overfeed, making their babies obese and overweight. Such extra fat may be very difficult for the child to lose in later years. By contrast, breastfed babies can almost never be overfed.

Deciding whether to Breastfeed or Bottlefeed

You and your partner can take all the foregoing pros and cons into account in reaching your decision on the method to use for feeding your baby. We suggest that you hold breastfeeding as an option as long as possible, to see how you feel right after birth. Doing so takes little or no extra effort.

You may want to combine the methods, in which case you will be deciding which method will be the main one rather than your only one. However, to get breastfeeding established, you should make it the method for about the first six weeks of your baby's life, and then continue to use breastfeeding as your main method (with your breast milk either consumed by the baby or expressed into bottles at intervals of no more than every six to eight hours).

You may benefit from attending a meeting of mothers who are feeding at breast and who have babies of all ages. Your prenatal class teacher can help, or you can seek out the local La Leche League chapter (see Appendix A).

Breast Care

Starting four to eight weeks before your baby is due, take about five minutes a day to massage your nipples and breasts. Doing this readies your breasts for nursing effectively and comfortably. Even if you plan to bottlefeed, follow the massage and other breast-care steps explained here. They will help head off breast discomfort and nipple soreness through the last months of pregnancy and the first weeks after your baby arrives.

A convenient time to carry out this daily massage is right after taking a bath, when your hands and body are clean. You'll need to have these supplies on hand: cotton balls (in a closed container), a skin cream or oil (La Leche suggests safflower oil, available very inexpensively in supermarkets), a hand brush, and if you wish, an additional ointment to use on your nipples (pure lanolin, A & D Ointment, or other breast cream).

Breast Massage

Carry out your daily five-minute routine of breast massage as follows.

Draw out the nipples: Working on the nipples helps to condition them for nursing and toughens them to help avoid later soreness.

If you haven't already, wash your hands thoroughly and clean under the nails with a hand brush. Sit comfortably with your trunk upright.

1. Support your breast with one hand.
2. With the thumb and forefinger of the other hand, grasp the nipple at its base, pulling gently, and roll it between your fingers.
3. Move your thumb and finger around the nipple, repeating step 2 until you have gone all around it.
4. Repeat for the other breast.

Massage the breast: Doing this massage improves circulation and eases engorgement of the breasts, which may occur in your last weeks of pregnancy. It also helps relieve congestion of the breasts after your baby is born.

Start by putting a few drops of skin cream or oil on your palms and rubbing them together.

1. Place one hand flat against your chest above one breast. Put your other hand on top of the first.
2. Slide your hands apart so that your fingers point downward, and encircle the breast from underneath, while your thumbs move together across the top of the breast.
3. Move your thumbs and fingers toward each other until they slide off the breast.
4. Repeat this massage ten times on each breast.

Apply ointment around the nipples: Rubbing ointment or oil into the areola (the area around the nipple) replaces natural skin oils and keeps the nipple supple.

Gently rub the ointment into the areola and the sides of the nipple, but avoid rubbing any ointment into the nipple duct openings.

Expressing colostrum: Colostrum appears on the nipples of some women in the later months of pregnancy. If you produce it early like this, you can relieve any pressure it may cause and clean it off your nipples with a cotton ball as described below.

After the baby's birth, you can express colostrum or milk in this manner in order to:

- facilitate the flow of milk as you start a feeding,
- tempt the infant onto the breast,
- relieve the initial distention of the breast at feeding time, so that the baby can more easily grasp the nipple and areola,
- express your milk into a clean bottle (to be refrigerated for a later bottlefeeding), or
- relieve any uncomfortable fullness you feel in the breasts when away from the baby.

Discuss this technique with your care-giver. Some prenatal care-givers think it's unimportant to express colostrum in this way during pregnancy.

1. Support the breast with one hand.
2. Gently place the pads of the thumb and forefinger of your other hand on the upper and lower edge of the areola. Stretch the areola as you push back against the breast.
3. Press your thumb and forefinger together and release.
4. Reposition your thumb and forefinger at several locations around the areola, and at each repeat steps 2 and 3, continuing around until you have completed a full circle.
5. Use a clean cotton ball to remove any colostrum that may have accumulated on the nipple.
6. Repeat steps 1 through 5 for the other breast.

Flat or Inverted Nipples

Some women have flat or inverted nipples that need special preparation for breastfeeding because they don't project out from the breast even when stimulated. Almost all such women can develop their nipples during pregnancy and can breastfeed successfully. Here's how.

Preparing flat nipples for breastfeeding: An adaptation of the breast massage exercise for drawing out the nipples usually proves effective with flat nipples. Do this as part of your daily breast massage routine:

1. Supporting your breast with one hand.
2. With the thumb and forefinger of the other hand, grasp the nipple at its base by pressing in firmly.

3. Pull the thumb and forefinger apart to stretch the nipple center and make it easier for the tip to stand out.
4. Move your thumb and forefinger around the nipple, stretching it in each position as described in step 3, until you've gone all around.

After a number of days, when the nipple begins to project more readily, you can grasp the nipple at its base, pull it gently, and roll it between your thumb and forefinger. Do this pulling and rolling with your hand going all around the nipple, first on one breast and then on the other.

Preparing inverted nipples for breastfeeding: In rare cases of fully inverted nipples, the nipple turns inward instead of outward when the areola is pressed between thumb and forefinger.

But even these and less completely inverted nipples can often be developed into outward-projecting nipples. This is done by wearing special breast shields during pregnancy, starting in the third month. At the outset they are used for a few hours a day, with their use being gradually extended up to eight hours a day.

These breast shields fit unobtrusively inside a bra. They consist of an outer and inner plastic cup fitting over the end of your breast. They are small and light. The inner one fits right over your skin and has a hole in the center for the gradually protruding nipple. The outer cup fits over the inner one and protects the nipple from chafing on your clothes.

Wearing breast shields for several months should remedy flat and even completely inverted nipples. Shields that are sound in design are available with complete instructions from La Leche International (see Appendix A).

Other Preparation for Your Nipples

A few other simple actions taken through the day will further help make the nipples less tender.

• When you dry yourself after bathing, rub each nipple gently with a soft terrycloth towel.
• For several hours a day, if you can, let your nipples rub against your clothing without protection (either by not wearing a bra or wearing a nursing bra with the panels open or an old bra with the centers cut out).

- Leave your nipples exposed to the air for as many minutes a day as you find practical.

- If workable, expose your nipples and breasts to the sunlight, but be extremely careful not to let them get sunburned.

Essentials of Breastfeeding

When and How to Start

You should start breastfeeding as soon as possible after you give birth. Having your brand-new baby cuddle with you skin-to-skin and start to suck at your breast can be one of the really important experiences of life—for the baby, for you, and for your partner.

Ideally, this will happen just minutes after the birth, even before you deliver the placenta. The baby's sucking can help strengthen the last contractions for expelling the placenta. It also will help to cut down your after-birth bleeding and assist the involution of your uterus.

Your baby even then starts to get your colostrum, with its antibodies for resistance to disease and for protection against allergies.

Breastfeeding at the Hospital or Birth Center

If you're having a hospital birth and you want to breastfeed, try to get complete rooming-in during the entire time you'll be in the hospital. With full rooming-in your baby's crib will stay right in your hospital room virtually all the time. In this way, it will be easier for you to breastfeed the baby at will, and there will be less chance that the baby will be fed supplementary water or formula.

If your baby must stay in the hospital nursery, ask your physician to leave strict orders that your baby is not to have any liquids besides your breast milk. If your doctor somehow can't do so, be polite but very persistent in telling the staff that you want your baby to have only your own breast milk.

Be as firm as you need to be about your determination to breastfeed in the hospital, because your milk might not come in well if your baby doesn't feed vigorously; your colostrum and milk are beyond question the best and only needed food for your baby's health.

In out-of-hospital birth centers, professionals are typically very much in favor of breastfeeding. During the relatively short time you'll be at the birth center, they will see to it that you have enough time to apply what you have learned in classes and get feeding established.

Feeding the Baby

Positions for feeding: Right after birth, your baby can breastfeed in any position that is comfortable for you. You can lie on your back, propped up, with the baby lying tummy down on your chest, mouth to your nipple. Or you can lie on your side with the baby lying on the bed with you and guide the nipple to the baby's mouth. Or you can sit upright, holding the baby's head in the crook of your elbow, and guide the nipple to baby's mouth while cuddling the baby against you.

After the baby is a few days old, you'll probably use the sitting-upright position for most feedings. A rocking chair can be especially soothing for this. You might want to do night feedings in bed, lying on your side.

The setting for breastfeeding: Breastfeed in a setting that's very peaceful and soothing for you and the baby. Too much noise, glare, and motion can distract the baby from feeding.

Peaceful surroundings also make it easier for your "let-down" reflex to work and start your milk flowing. The let-down reflex is a physical response to the start of feeding, but it often takes a little learning and familiarity with the nursing process. Even if your let-down doesn't become apparent to you for some weeks, you can reassure yourself that your baby is getting enough milk by its swallowing sounds. The reflex occurs for some mothers with just knowing the baby is due to start nursing, or with the baby's touch on the breasts or nipples. It can also arise when hearing the baby cry, or even someone else's baby. You may feel it as a tingling and heavy sensation that comes over your breasts, and that brings your nipples erect and starts milk flowing for the feeding.

Although you need the right emotional stimulus to trigger your let-down reflex, it is a physical reaction. The hormone oxytocin is released into your bloodstream by the pituitary gland, causing cells around the milk glands to contract, squeezing the milk into sacs near the nipple.

Getting the baby to take the nipple correctly: When you start a feeding, guide your baby to take the nipple by holding the baby's searching mouth near the nipple. With a finger, gently stroke the baby's cheek on the side nearest the nipple, so that its head turns to find it. A few drops of colostrum or milk expressed on the nipple may help. After a few days or perhaps weeks, when you touch a nipple to the cheek, the baby will turn to it right away.

Make sure the baby takes the nipple and areola completely into its mouth. In this fashion the baby's sucking, which is actually more of a biting motion, will fully press the milk out of the milk sacs and through the milk ducts. If the baby nurses only on the outer nipple, he or she may not get enough food and the nipples will very likely become sore.

Nursing time: Your baby will probably suck at uneven rates, sometimes going fast, other times slowly, and still other times just resting with lips on nipple before starting up again.

In a lull after the baby has fed for some minutes on one breast, shift the baby over to the other. Shift also when you want to relieve a sense of fullness in the other breast. Some minutes later you can shift the baby back to the first breast. This shifting back and forth helps develop the baby's eye coordination, some authorities think.

Babies have been found to get most of their food in the first eight to ten minutes of a feeding. The sucking that continues on past ten to twelve minutes or more may serve important purposes in the baby's emotional development.

The baby may drowse off a few minutes into the feeding. When this happens, gently stir the baby awake by talking softly or by lightly stroking a cheek. On waking up, the baby may feed quite actively for a while. These cycles of drowsing and then waking and eating may occur several times in a feeding.

In view of the baby's needs for leisurely dining and long sucking, let each feeding run up to fifteen, twenty, or thirty minutes and more in length, insofar as possible. That can be hard in the early days, when the baby is eating as often as every two hours. Intervals of four to six hours, at least between night feedings, usually develop after just a few weeks. And the value of long, leisurely feedings in the earliest weeks are substantial for the baby's physical and emotional development and could be a factor in having a contented infant and perhaps lifelong emotional strength as well.

Burping the baby: After the baby has fed for some minutes and seems to be getting full, take it off the breast by inserting your little finger in the corner of its mouth to break the suction that has formed. Next, move the baby so that its head and tummy rest against your shoulder. Then pat it gently on the back for a few minutes. In time, the position and the pats may bring up a burp you can clearly hear. It consists mostly of air swallowed while crying before the feeding or in getting established on the nipple.

Another burping position is to hold the baby lying tummy down across your knees and pat gently on its back. If the baby doesn't burp, just resume nursing. Breastfed babies swallow little air compared to bottlefed babies.

How to tell when the baby has had enough: Long, leisurely feedings like those described above provide babies with just the right amount to eat in almost all cases. Very much the same factors that worked between mother and baby to give enough nourishment before birth are still working after the birth: the baby naturally consumes all it needs, and the mother's system naturally produces enough to meet those needs, providing the mother's diet is adequate.

The baby's general contentment is a sign that he or she has had enough to eat. In the baby's natural behavior, he or she will cry and fuss when hungry and be quiet when full.

One indirect way of checking is to look at the urinary output of a breastfed baby. Some mothers say it's likely that a new baby is getting enough to eat if it has at least six to eight very wet diapers a day. (Sometimes it's hard to be sure how wet disposables are.)

Over longer time periods you'll naturally gauge whether the baby is eating enough by its growth and weight gain. Weight gains of babies who are completely healthy and well fed vary enormously. Your caregiver can help you judge your own infant's development. In their first few days of extrauterine life, infants lose 7–10 percent of their weight at birth due to excretion of stored fluids. Typically, the weight the baby had at birth is usually regained in ten days to three weeks after birth. After its birth weight is regained, it should gain one-half pound per week (2 or more pounds per month). One pound per month is too little; four or more pounds, too much. An even better guide is whether the baby is generally healthy, happy, active, and alert.

When to feed the baby? In keeping with the naturally self-regulating rhythms of breastfeeding, feed your new baby when he or she cries and fusses, which is usually an expression of hunger. That may be every two or three hours round the clock in the beginning.

Gradually, those times when the baby is hungry will stretch to about every four hours through the day and four to six hours or more overnight. At times the intervals between feedings will be uneven—as little as two hours or as long as six hours. But the normal eating pattern will usually be quite regular.

No other food: Through at least the first six months of life, when breastfeeding is proceeding well, your baby needs to eat or drink nothing besides your breast milk to get all that is required for good health.

You can have a clean nursing bottle of boiled plain water at hand to give as a kind of pacifier, but it's not at all necessary. Besides breast milk, the American Academy of Pediatrics recommends no so-called solid foods before the age of five or six months. Until then, the baby's system hasn't matured enough to digest them.

And as for vitamins, the baby needs no supplement. However, many pediatricians advise providing supplements of vitamins A, C, and D.

How to Increase Your Milk Supply

Your milk is produced very largely during the feeding itself by the milk-secreting glands deep inside your breast. Very little of it is made ahead of time and stored. It's almost all made to order and completely fresh.

Don't worry about running out of milk as your baby grows bigger and hungrier. The baby's own eating stimulates the development of more milk. To produce more milk, simply let the baby nurse more.

It is important to make sure you're drinking enough liquids yourself. Some mothers find that their milk flows better if they drink a big glass of water or juice just before they give baby a feeding, or if they have a glass at hand to sip.

Drink about as much liquid as you did during pregnancy. Aim for eight tall glasses of water a day plus another four glasses of milk, unless you have your equivalent of a quart of milk a day in products like yogurt or cottage cheese instead. And if you still feel thirsty at times, drink still more liquids.

If you want to keep your milk supply growing in pace with the baby's growth, there's one thing to avoid. Don't start giving your baby occasional bottles of formula instead of breast milk before the sixth week, or an occasional dish of solid baby food—at least not before the age of four to six months. However, with a young baby, if for some reason you must miss a feeding, formula is always preferable to juice.

Your baby will take less at the breast if it's filling up on other foods. And eating less will cut down on the amount of milk you produce in response. If you are not careful, your milk production may then decline before you really want to stop nursing. From time immemorial, babies have been weaned and breast milk curtailed by gradually intro-ducing the child to other foods.

However, some mothers find that they can give their babies an occasional bottle of formula once their breastfeeding has become firmly established, after at least several months. These mothers say they succeeded in doing this because of their determination to continue breastfeeding.

Your Diet While Breastfeeding

To satisfy the nutritional needs of both yourself and your baby while nursing, eat the same kinds and proportions of foods that you did during pregnancy (as explained in Chapter 4). It is recommended that you add 500 calories and 40 grams of protein a day while nursing. To accomplish this, increase what you eat by these amounts:

• With high-protein foods, eat five servings a day instead of four.
• With whole-grain foods or fruits (or starchy vegetables), eat two additional servings a day.

In addition, nutritionists usually suggest that you continue taking iron tablets (30 to 60 milligrams a day) and vitamin B_9 (400 to 800 micrograms a day).

You could also ask your baby's health-care-giver or pediatrician if other adjustments or supplements to your diet might be helpful.

How Long Should You Continue Breastfeeding?

How long to continue nursing is largely up to you to decide. Most of your immunities have been passed on to your baby by about the fifth or sixth month, and the baby's system can increasingly digest other foods from about then on.

Some mothers, though, go on nursing for the emotional well-being of their children and further transfer of immunities and nutrition until eight or nine months, and a few mothers continue up to and sometimes long after the first birthday.

Encouragement and Help from Other Mothers

You probably can get information and help on any aspect of breast-feeding right in your own locale, in your regular prenatal classes. In addition, you are sure to find experienced and sympathetic members of the La Leche League right in your vicinity. So dedicated are League members that some of them even breastfeed babies of other mothers incapacitated by sudden emergencies. The League has more than 4,000 chapters worldwide.

Essentials of Bottlefeeding

When and How to Start

If you're having a hospital birth, you can begin bottlefeeding almost as soon as your baby is born. Hospitals carry out bottlefeeding as part of their normal procedures. (And they often give water in the nursery as the first feeding to check for anomalies of the esophagus.) Simply let your care-givers know, when you enter the hospital or before, that you want your baby bottlefed from birth on and that you prefer not to breastfeed.

If you do choose bottlefeeding starting at birth, discuss with your care-giver whether you will be given a hormonal injection to dry up your milk supply (these are usually thought to be most effective when given right after birth). And if so, which hormonal preparation will be injected? Ask your care-giver to explain any possibly injurious effects. You may be asked to sign a patient information sheet indicating you have received the information.

On the other hand, you may choose to breastfeed your baby for at least the first few days. There are three main reasons for doing so:

- to give your baby the benefit of a number of important immunities transmitted in your colostrum and early milk,
- to have the experience of breastfeeding, and
- to have your milk dry up naturally rather than by hormone injections (you would simply give bottles of formula at more frequent feedings).

If you start in this way, you could naturally go on with breastfeeding for as many weeks or months as you wish before converting to bottles.

Formulas, Bottles, and Nipples

Breast-milk substitutes used for bottlefeeding babies are called "infant formulas" because they are artificially compounded, from either a cow's-milk base or a soybean base. You may have heard friends use the trade names of some of these, such as Enfamil, Similac, Isomil, SMA, and Prosobee. Formulas approach the composition of human milk in various respects but none exactly duplicates it. Major respects in which formulas and human milk are compared include type of protein, ratio of protein to fat content, amino acid content, and proportion of the valuable lactose form of sugar.

Pediatricians usually advise that selecting a formula for a specific baby should be left to them or other professionals because so many technical questions are involved in the choice. If your baby has been started on formula feedings after a hospital birth, you will be told which formula to use. On leaving the hospital, you'll probably be given a small supply along with a few bottles and nipples. Nurses at the hospital will tell you how to use these when they are explaining ways of taking care of your baby generally.

Some babies develop allergies or colic with stomach aches on a formula and then need to have a different formula prescribed by their physician.

Advice on any supplements of vitamins and minerals for your baby should also come from your pediatrician or other care-giver. Such supplements need to be specified in relation to the vitamins and minerals already contained in the specific formula recommended.

Plastic bottles that can be boiled might be better than glass bottles, because plastic is unbreakable. Moreover, should you use bottles for storing your own breast milk, plastic may be preferable. Certain ingredients in breast milk stick to the walls of glass bottles (and thus never get to the baby) but do not adhere to plastic.

Plastic liner bottles are especially convenient. They are cylindrical in shape but with open bottoms, and are lined with pouches of thin-walled, flexible plastic which are discarded and replaced after each use. The pouch collapses as the baby drinks, and the baby swallows less air as a result.

As for bottle nipples, you can get either the conventional straight-up type or irregularly shaped ones that are designed for sound tooth and jaw development and are endorsed by orthodontists.

In the past, pediatricians almost universally recommended that all nursing bottles and nipples, as well as all spoons and other implements used in preparing formula, be sterilized by boiling them in water for a specified time. Today many pediatricians advise that it's sufficient just to wash them thoroughly in very hot water (or in a dishwasher). They also recommend keeping filled bottles in the refrigerator. Request your care-giver's instructions on sterilizing or washing and refrigerating.

Don't keep partially consumed formula for any length of time. Throw it away rather than trying to use it up. It may have developed enough harmful germs to give the baby digestive troubles.

How to Bottlefeed Your Baby

For bottlefeeding, use essentially the same positions for holding and cuddling the baby, the same peaceful setting, and the same way of burping your baby as you would for breastfeeding. You may need to burp the baby long and often—babies often swallow more air when bottlefed than when breastfed.

After holding the baby for five minutes or so on one arm, wait for the baby to pause and then shift her or him over to the other arm. Make the shift in much the same way as you would from one breast to the other. Doing this helps develop the baby's eye coordination.

Never leave the baby alone, eating from a bottle propped up by a pillow or cloth with no one else around. The baby might choke on the milk or breathe some of it into the lungs.

How Much and How Often to Bottlefeed Your Baby

Your baby's system will naturally tell you when it needs to be fed and when it has eaten enough to be healthy and content. Your pediatrician, pediatric nurse-practitioner, or other care-giver can tell you what a maximum feeding amount would be for the baby's age. Have that maximum amount ready in the bottle, but don't try to make baby eat all of it. Your baby will stop eating when full, and then probably doze off to sleep.

Give the baby feedings when he or she gets hungry and tells you so. Avoid holding to a fixed schedule, like every two hours or every four hours. Especially in the first few days, the baby may eat at somewhat irregular intervals—two hours between feedings one time, three hours or so another time. After several months, the baby will be eating on a fairly regular schedule but should be allowed to vary somewhat from the usual time for an occasional feeding.

12

❦

Preparing Your Family and Home for the Baby

Childbearing families today have more options open to them than ever before, including choices about the roles to be played by the people close to them—children, parents, other relatives, and even good friends. You and your partner are the directors, and you can decide how things will be done. The people you select to participate may take on roles very different from traditional ones.

Preparing Family Members

With parents, in-laws, or any other relatives especially close to you or your partner, be clear and firm about the kind of birth that you have chosen. If parents or other authority-figure relatives criticize and give unwanted advice—particularly about ways of birthing unfamiliar to them—try to be considerate. Try not to respond emotionally. Instead, make them aware that you have carefully studied and investigated every aspect and that your decision is informed and intelligent. Also, be sure enough of yourself to be practical and accept any needed help, monetary or otherwise, they may offer without feeling compromised.

At a birth center (and certainly at a home birth), you can easily have one or two adult relatives with you or in a nearby room through labor. In the latter choice, they can come in and talk to you at points during labor and right after the birth—or can even be in the same room with you at birth, if you wish. Occasionally hospitals also offer this option.

In particular, the grandparents of your newborn—your own parents or your partner's—might be a positive help through labor and birth. Some childbearing women find that having one or more grandparents present for the birth brings everyone a very special satisfaction.

Or, if it would be helpful to you, one or two very close friends could join in the experience, rather than relatives.

However, make sure that each person there knows realistically what labor and birth are like and can be of assistance to you. Ideally, they would attend the prenatal classes on labor and see some films or tapes of birth.

No person with a cold or other contagious illness should be allowed to be present.

Deciding on Roles for Your Children

What role you want your children to play is an intensely personal question. At one extreme, a child would be told only as much as necessary, without evading questions. Answers can be simple but honest (for example, only that the baby was growing in mother's uterus or womb, or a special place, and that it would come out into the world in ways the child is too young to understand just now).

At the other extreme, you would tell the child in understandable but accurate terms how the baby was growing. In this way your child is prepared to be with you and your partner during the labor and perhaps also actually at the birth, and to join with you in bonding with the baby.

Any role at or between these extremes can be a constructive experience for your child. Just be sure to give your children special attention from the beginning of your pregnancy. Consider the special personal and emotional advantages for you and your child if he or she attends the birth or is nearby. Plan carefully for the child's role, and then talk it over in advance. Above all, don't just automatically assume what that role will be or just let it happen.

The special attention needed by children: You'll want to give your children special attention once you learn you are pregnant. They will need extra love and attention even if they don't show it. This includes praise when called for, explanations when they show curiosity, and sometimes jobs to do to make them feel a part of this adventure. All of these things will avoid hurt feelings, hostility, and the sense that they have been left out or replaced by someone more important.

In these ways you may even help prevent emotional problems in later life.

Here are some suggestions for meeting children's needs during your pregnancy:

- *Treat the event as a maturing one:*   Put yourself in a new mindset about your son or daughter. He or she is not just the baby any more, but is becoming a big brother or big sister. Start remembering to give special love and praise so your child will not feel pushed aside or forgotten by you and your partner. At the same time, communicate in words and actions how much you treasure her or him as your very own child who goes on getting bigger, stronger, and more helpful and self-reliant than when a baby. Remind your child that, although a new baby whom you will also love is on the way, you have loved him or her longer.

- *Explain what's happening and what to expect:*   As early as possible, tell your child in a warm, quiet, loving talk that the baby has begun growing and will arrive at a time in the future, which you might indicate by the season of the year. Relate the baby's expected birth to the child's own age at that time. Give some explanation for how the baby's life began in terms the youngster can understand. Many expectant parents today find it best to outline the actual events in a brief, relaxed, matter-of-fact way. There are many books for children on pregnancy and birth (see Appendix B).

  Use whatever explanation you and your partner prefer. You might supplement it with drawings or photographs. You can use the illustrations in this book, for example. Your library probably also has a number of appropriate books.

  But most important, start early to make a family team for bringing the baby into your home and the world. That will prevent the child from feeling left out when you, your partner, and others talk about and plan for the new arrival.

- *Spend regular special times with the child:*   A few times a day for several minutes, give the youngster your complete undivided attention and love. Do this at about the same hour each day, such as in the morning after getting everyone off to work or school, after lunch in the early afternoon, or at bedtime. A few minutes can be enough to convey the sense that your youngster can still count on your complete devotion. They show that you can still love him or her just as much while also loving the baby. They start habitual times of special closeness that can go on long after the baby arrives.

- *Let the child share and help as part of the family team:*   Sharing in the baby's growth and helping get ready for the baby can be fostered by letting your boy or girl feel your abdomen as it grows, and by pointing out the baby's movements. Also, let your child hear the baby's heartbeat by putting an ear to your abdomen. Some careproviders will welcome your child at prenatal visits and let the child listen through the stethoscope.

Include him or her in talking about plans for the baby—where the crib will go, where you'll put the baby's clothes, how you'll give the baby a bath, and what you'll do about the baby's diapers. Let the youngster help, as with folding crib blankets or moving furniture.

- *Mention the child often in talk with friends:* Refer to him or her frequently when discussing the baby with friends and relatives. Talk about how well your child understands and helps, and how you love him all the more. Remind friends and relatives that when they think of getting things to give the baby, they should also get a little something for these wonderful siblings of the baby.

- *Give things to the child when getting things for the baby:* When you bustle about getting all the things needed for the baby, draw your child into the planning and decision-making. At the same time, try to get some things for her or him, too. Even little things, given with love, will help your son or daughter feel included and still cherished.

These efforts won't always keep your older child or children from feeling and showing some resentment of the new baby's approaching arrival. But they'll help lay a foundation for developing a healthy acceptance and love for the new little brother or sister in time.

Class Sessions for Your Children

Classes are now given expressly for the children of expectant parents. You can find out whether any are available in your locale by asking when you inquire about prenatal classes. These sessions for children are almost always given in conjunction with prenatal classes for adults.

Some programs of prenatal classes offer a series of classes specifically for mothers who have previously given birth, and may provide sessions designed for older children. Sessions for the children may include features like listening to the heartbeats of their baby sister or brother with a stethoscope, finding out how other children feel about getting a new baby sister or brother, and having an advance birthday party with cake, candles, and ice cream to celebrate the birth early.

Class sessions at birth centers often include other features for children who are prepared to be present for the birth. Explanations of the birth process may be given. Color films or videotapes of actual births may also be shown, with the parents' approval. These give the children an idea of what to expect when they are present at the birth, in order to help further prepare them for the event.

Children Present at the Birth

Increasing numbers of expectant parents today like the idea of having their children present at the birth. Almost all hospital birth settings exclude children during labor and birth; even so, if interested, you should ask.

You can usually arrange to have your child (or children) near you for the birth by choosing either a birth center or home birth, where it is a common arrangement. There, the decision on whether to have your child present is left entirely up to you and the child.

It is widely thought that, if the child and parents are willing and are prepared, having the child present may help the boy or girl feel more attached to the baby and to the family as a whole. Some informal studies suggest that children present at the birth show less hostility to a new baby brother or sister.

Flexibility regarding children (and other family members) represents a distinct advantage of birth conducted at a birth center or at home. In either setting your child does not need to be separated from you and from the momentous family occasion of birth. At the same time, however, the child need not be at your side through the whole experience. The child can be in another room, being looked after by an adult relative or friend through all parts of the labor and birth. Yet the child can see you whenever desirable, and can join you as part of the family right after the birth.

If you're using a birth center and want your child present for the birth, you would usually be advised to take the following steps:

1. Bring the child with you for at least some of your early checkups at the center so that she or he will feel at home there.

2. Prepare your child to be present at the birth in ways the center staff members recommend, such as attending a special prenatal class session.

3. Have an adult come along to the center to look after your child, since your partner will be busy working as your support person through labor and birth.

Arrangements like these are advisable for a home birth as well.

Getting Set for the Baby

In addition to getting your family ready for the baby's arrival, you need to get your home ready as well. Here's what you'll need in the way of furniture and equipment, and clothes and supplies.

ESSENTIAL BABY FURNITURE AND EQUIPMENT

1. ☐ Crib or other baby bed—one of the following:

   Crib: A full-size crib is the most common choice for a new baby's bed, as it can be used for several years and is durable and safe. It measures 53 inches long by 30½ inches wide, and must meet federal safety standards and be labeled accordingly.

   Folding crib, or "portacrib":   Measuring about 39 by 25 inches, a folding crib can be handy in limited space or for traveling. It also converts to a small playpen, and can be outfitted with mattresses, pads, sheets, and bumpers in sizes to fit.

   Cradle or bassinet: A small cradle or bassinet is snug and close-fitting for the newborn baby, but will be outgrown after the baby is only three or four months old.

   Bureau drawer (or similar sturdy box or basket):   Any of these should prove satisfactory once you pad it along the bottom and sides, and put it on a solid, secure surface off the floor.

2. Bedding and blankets, which should include:

   ☐ 1 firm, waterproof mattress; must fit snugly against crib sides

   ☐ 1 crib bumper (inner padding to keep baby from bumping against the inside railings) with ties or snaps to keep it in place

   ☐ 2 mattress pads, either cotton flannelette or cotton-quilted; fitted style; should have a rubberized middle layer

   ☐ 3 fitted sheets, cotton knit or cotton-polyester knit

   ☐ 3–4 waterproof protective pads to place under baby's head and bottom

   ☐ 4–6 receiving blankets (lightweight flannelette)

   ☐ 2 crib blankets (thermal type or acrylic may be preferable as they are light in weight)

   Optional bedding items include:

   ☐ 1 mobile toy (stimulates baby's vision and captures baby's attention) that can be fastened to crib frame

3. Bath equipment, which may include:

   ☐ 3 baby-size washcloths

   ☐ 2 ordinary, soft bath towels, terrycloth or knit; towels with hoods aren't needed

   ☐ mild soap

   ☐ 1 box of cotton balls (for cleaning eyes, ears, and nose; do *not* use cotton-tipped swabs; keep cotton balls in a covered container)

   ☐ 1 emery nail-filing board or blunt-tipped nail scissors

   ☐ 1 baby comb and brush set

   Optional bath equipment items include:

   ☐ 1 baby-size plastic bathtub (or use the kitchen sink instead; if you do, make sure it is well cleaned and lined with a towel or cloth diaper to prevent slipping)

   ☐ 1 small tray (for convenience in holding baby's bath and toilet articles; a baking pan may be used instead)

   ☐ 1 box cornstarch (some families prefer this natural substance over talcum powder for the baby)

4. Feeding equipment, which should include:

   If you will be breastfeeding—

   ☐ 1–2 nursing bottles (1 is enough if you are using plastic bottles with disposable linings)

   ☐ 2 rubber nipples (ones of special orthodontic design, like NUK brand nipples, are often recommended)

   Or, if you will be bottlefeeding—

   ☐ 8–10 nursing bottles if you are using those without plastic liners, or 2–3 bottles if you are using those with plastic liners (8-ounce bottles are handiest for feeding)

   ☐ 8–10 nipples if using non-plastic-liner bottles, or 5 nipples if using those with plastic liners (ones of orthodontic design are often advised)

5. ☐ Infant auto seat (required by law in some states, New York among them; police stations in some of these states will provide seats on loan)

6. Health-care equipment, which should include:

   ☐ rectal thermometer

☐ petroleum jelly

☐ anti-fever medication (such as baby acetaminophen)

☐ rubber ear syringe or infant nasal aspirator

☐ adhesive bandages of various sizes

☐ tweezers

☐ antiseptic for minor first aid

☐ ointment to prevent or treat diaper rash (types suggested include those containing a zinc-oxide or cod-liver-oil base)

☐ vaporizer or humidifier (highly recommended)

7. Other desirable equipment:

☐ baby-carrier sling to carry the baby against the chest

☐ baby carriage or stroller (not really needed in baby's earliest weeks)

☐ framed backpack carrier after 4 or 5 months of age

ESSENTIAL BABY SUPPLIES AND CLOTHES

1. *Diapers,* using one or more of these options:

☐ 4–6 dozen or more disposable diapers, newborn size (you'll use 8 to 12 or more a day); some parents prefer the type with elasticized tucks, which prevent leaking. Follow directions on the box for use and disposal. Even if you use disposable diapers, a half-dozen or more cloth diapers are handy for burp towels, bibs, etc.

Or, if you plan to launder your own diapers—

☐ 4 dozen cloth diapers. Some parents prefer the prefolded, gauze type of diapers, and a few others prefer diapers that are also contour-shaped; be sure to wash before using. For laundering, first shake off any fecal material from used diapers into the toilet and then store used diapers in a large covered plastic pail half-filled with a solution of borax or bleach; launder separately from your family's clothes, using a small amount of mild detergent or soap and rinsing well to avoid any residue that could be irritating to the baby. Borax or bleach can be added to the rinse cycle, but fabric softeners used to excess may make diapers less absorbent; drying in automatic dryers softens and fluffs diapers.

☐ 4 double-lock diaper safety pins for cloth diapers (2 for use, 2 spares; be sure to get the double-lock pins that can't open by accident; disposable diapers have self-stick tabs and don't need pinning)

Or—

☐ use a diaper service that delivers cloth diapers and picks up soiled ones, usually once a week.

2. ☐ 4–6 pairs of *waterproof pants* if you are using cloth diapers. Get the smallest size for your newborn baby, which will still probably be too big around the thighs. Choose the lightweight nylon types, which are cooler and which last longer than vinyl types, and get a pull-on rather than snap-on type, since pull-ons are easier to use and last longer.

3. ☐ 6–8 *undershirts,* all cotton or cotton-polyester fabric; 6-months size is small enough since the baby grows rapidly and the shirts shrink. Some parents think the short-sleeve, snap-front style is easiest to use with newborns; other styles are over-the-head and long-sleeve or sleeveless. One-piece underwear with crotch snaps are very popular. Disposable diapers make it possible to forego waterproof pants for them. Underwear sets are also available in two pieces.

4. ☐ 6–8 *outer garments* (stretch suits, sleeping bags, or nightgowns); 6-months or 12-months size. Stretch suits are widely used; make sure they're big enough so that the snap-closing crotch area is not tight, and that the feet are roomy enough for the baby's toes. Sleeping bags have front zippers and pouch-style closed ends to keep the baby's feet warm; some zippers are two-way for diaper-changing without taking off the entire bag; check for a cloth backing at the zipper top to protect the baby's neck from being pinched by the zipper. Nightgowns come with either open or drawstring-closed bottoms. Check garments for meeting federal flame-retardant standards for childrens' sleepwear.

5. ☐ 2–3 *outdoor outfits* (sweater-and-cap sets, buntings, or pram suits including sweater, cap, and leggings); 6-months or 12-months size; if you get the 12-months size, it may still fit through a second winter. Synthetic materials are preferable to wool because synthetics are usually less irritating to the baby's skin and launder easily.

Household and Social Arrangements to Make in Advance

Plan to reduce the demands on your time and energy through your last weeks of pregnancy and early months of caring for the baby. Make necessary arrangements at work, at home, and in your social life. At the same time, it is important to keep occupied in the last weeks of pregnancy.

What you'll do to decrease these demands depends on your specific situation. However, consider these suggestions:

- Get the things you'll need for the baby (as outlined earlier) three to four weeks before your due date.

- Finish early or postpone for six months or more any plans for extensive redecorating, renovating, or other major changes you want to make in your home. Try not to let your end-of-pregnancy nesting instinct tire you. At this time it's easy to "bite off more than you can chew."

- Mobilize grandparents or other relatives or congenial friends to help with the housework, meals, shopping, and other chores after the baby arrives.

- If you're planning an early return to work, begin interviewing caretakers for the baby. If you plan to feed at breast, be sure to sound out applicants' feelings about this.

- If you already have a child or children, set up some advance or standby baby-sitting plans with congenial relatives, friends, or reliable teenage sitters. Also, if any of the children are about age 6 or older, seek their cooperation ahead of time to take on some regular household chores. Explain that this will give you more time to spend with them and the baby.

- Find out about some household cleaning services and mother's-helper services you could call on if needed. Information about such services is often available through prenatal class teachers.

Don't be surprised if, in the midst of preparing for the baby, you find you have intense urges to tackle ambitious home projects, with energy bursts to match. Expectant women often get such feelings near the end of their pregnancy and set off in a flurry of activity, repainting rooms, fixing or buying furniture, or refurbishing the entire family wardrobe.

Emotions like these arise so commonly that they're sometimes thought to result from a kind of nesting instinct or impulse. Take care not to start endeavors that are too ambitious and not really practical. Instead, capitalize on all that energy to do things that will be genuinely useful in saving you time and exertion after the baby arrives.

Added Arrangements to Make for a Home Birth

If you are planning a home birth, you'll have more to think about in terms of preparing the room where you will labor and give birth. It should be close to a bathroom for both your convenience and the care-giver's. The room should also be large enough for you to move around freely and to comfortably accommodate the family and friends who will attend the birth. A comfortable rocker or lounge chair may feel good to you in early labor.

Your care-giver will probably give you a list of items to have on hand. Have them ready well in advance of your due date. He or she will need a table close to the bed on which to place equipment and supplies. In general, the care-giver will bring along any necessary supplies.

A few basins or very clean buckets for waste will prove helpful, as well as plastic bags for double-wrapping the placenta. (If you plan to bury it, be sure to prepare a deep hole to prevent roving pets or other animals from digging it up.)

Lighting is important. Your care-giver will need one strong lamp to use for checking your genitalia after the birth. If you want soft, diffuse lighting for the labor and birth, indirect lamps that shine up toward the ceiling work well.

+

III

Birth and Early Parenting

13

᳁᳁᳁᳁᳁

Labor and Delivery– Giving Birth

Keeping occupied and feeling positive and relaxed should be your major aims as you approach your due date. Try not to become impatient. This is the time to complete any final preparations, in order to ease your first days at home with your baby. Remember, you have prepared yourself well and can continue calm and confident in what you're doing, right on through actually having your baby. Attend any labor rehearsal sessions your childbirth educators may provide.

The Last Weeks of Pregnancy

Lightening and Engagement

Lightening, or dropping, occurs when the baby settles downward into your upper pelvis (Figure 13.1). This can take place as early as two or three weeks before labor—especially if it is your first baby—or not until labor begins.

After lightening, you'll be able to take deep breaths more easily, because your lungs will have more room in which to expand. But there will be more pressure on your bladder and you will need to urinate more often. You may get aches in your legs at times, too, as the pressure of the baby's head affects the circulation to and from your legs.

Engagement, when the baby's head settles deeply into the pelvis, reaching certain bony prominences, the ischial spines, may—but not always—accompany lightening.

How You'll Feel

Your body systems will be working very hard by this time, and you may feel sluggish and awkward. On the other hand, some women feel a new surge of energy in the days immediately before labor. Make sure you get enough rest. Take daytime naps when you can and go

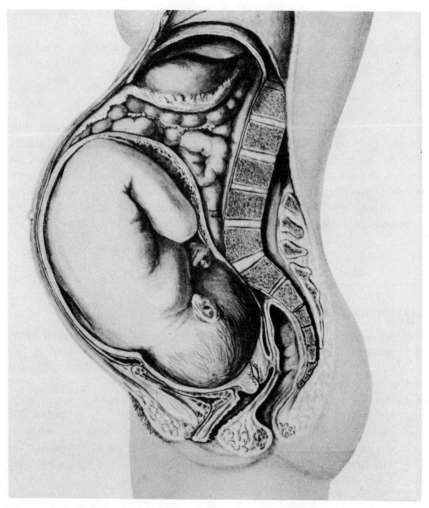

Figure 13.1. Before lightening

to bed earlier at night. Keep taking enough iron in your diet; lack of iron can cause anemia, a condition that makes you feel tired regardless of how much rest you get.

Most weight gain at the end of pregnancy goes to the baby, who typically adds a pound or more in the last weeks.

Emotionally, expectant women cope with three sets of feelings shortly before labor: impatience for labor to begin, uncertainty about how they will do through labor, and excited anticipation about seeing the baby.

Some women become slightly depressed at this time, whereas others

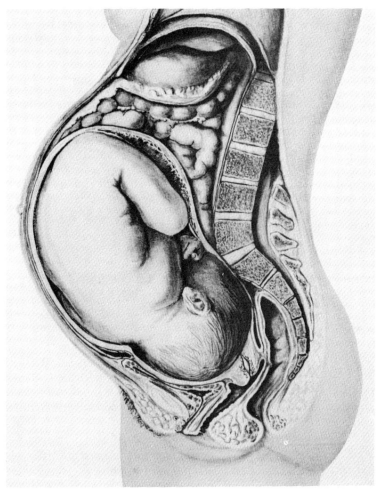

After lightening

feel elated. If you feel down or discouraged, try to keep occupied doing enjoyable things and making preparations for the baby's arrival. Spend time with other women who have had good pregnancy and birth experiences, and turn your thoughts in positive directions whenever you start worrying about what lies ahead; share your concerns with your prenatal education classmates and others who understand, the family you have selected to support you. You'll be seeing your provider weekly at this time; share your feelings in these last prenatal visits.

Also, check to make sure that your nutrition is good and you're getting enough to eat.

By all means, go right on with your breathing and body exercises every day as you've been doing for weeks now—with your support person whenever possible. Soon you'll be using those muscles and skills you've developed.

Choosing the Health-Care Provider for Your Baby

If you haven't done so already, it's very important now to decide on a professional who will provide health-care services for your baby after it's born. You and your partner should try not to rush into making this choice. Leave enough time to find and consider two or more possibilities, if you can.

In most instances, the health-care professional providing your maternity-care services through pregnancy and labor turns over responsibility for the baby right after birth. This is almost always the case at birth centers and hospitals. Birth centers customarily require you to arrange well before your due date for a pediatrician or professional in family practice to furnish care for your infant. In team practices, pediatric nurse practitioners may be available for newborn care, in some cases as an extension of birth center services.

Your birth care provider checks the baby through Apgar Scoring right at birth and is alert for any immediate problems in adjustment to the new environment.

Your baby's care-provider usually will examine the newborn within twenty-four hours after birth. If for any reason the pediatric care-provider you have chosen cannot see your baby soon after birth, hospitals or birth centers will usually have a staff or consultant pediatrician examine your baby before you leave for home. (There may be an additional fee for this examination.) The birth certificate, however, is filled out and signed by the physician or certified nurse-midwife who attended the mother through the labor and birth.

If you are having a home birth, be sure the baby's care-provider is aware of that fact in the event you need his or her services there.

Where to get suggestions: Research, investigate, and decide on a care-provider for your baby in the same way you did for yourself. By this point, you'll probably have three additional sources of suggestions for possible infant care-givers—the professional providing your maternity care, other expectant parents in your prenatal classes, and your childbirth educator.

Or, consult your usual family care-provider, neighbors, relatives, or friends. Should you be enrolled in a health maintenance organization (HMO) for your health-care insurance, a licensed practitioner to provide newborn health-care may already be selected for you.

After you've done some inquiring and narrowing down, interview the one or more professionals you're seriously considering for infant care before making your decision. Any sound professional should welcome such an interview. A checklist for these interviews appears below.

Some birth centers provide ongoing "new-family care" for mothers and infants that includes physical care as well as parenting classes or discussion groups.

CHECKLIST FOR SELECTING YOUR BABY'S CARE-PROVIDER

1. Type of practice (check one): _____
   - ☐ Individual; if so, whom can I reach when you're not available?
   - ☐ Group; if so, who gives us care for what/when? _____

2. Professional background (check one):
   - ☐ M.D.
     Board-certified in pediatrics? _____
   - ☐ D.O.
     Board-certified in pediatrics? _____
   - ☐ Nurse practitioner
     Physician(s) with whom associated in practice _____

3. Do you make house calls? ☐ yes ☐ no. Comments: _____

4. What are your Mon.–Fri. telephone hours? _____
   Can I get telephone advice in an emergency? ☐ Yes ☐ No. If yes, how? _____

---

5. In regular office examinations of a baby, what do you record and check on? □ weight, □ length (height), □ eating, □ sleeping, □ bowel movements, □ energy, □ general health, □ immunizations, □ emotional development, □ health or developmental problems, if any, □ problems we are having with the baby's care, if any.

6. What hospital(s) are you affiliated with, and which would be the one(s) to which you would have us take the baby if need arises?

___

7. Fees and payment: What are your fees for starting care of the baby (including examination soon after birth), if:

• the baby is normal and there are no complications?   ___

• there are complications, and the baby is not normal?   ___

What are your fees for regular care?

per office visit ___

per immunization ___

per house call ___

for special services (laboratory tests, special examinations, minor office treatment like stitches, etc.) ___

Notes: ___

Which health-care insurance coverage plans are acceptable for payment? ___

Will you accept payment directly from my insurance company? □ Yes □ No

Making Preparations

At some point in these latter weeks make your practical arrangements:

• Jot down the phone numbers of your care-giver, the birth center or hospital, and a standby helper or two on whom you could call.

• Arrange for people to look after children or pets if necessary.

• Plan the trip to the birth center or hospital. Be sure you know main and alternative routes and the time each route takes; also, provide for backup transportation methods, just in case.

• Arrange for photographs or a video tape of the labor and birth if you want (many expectant parents today think this is important). If you plan to do this, have an extra person who is not your labor partner do the picture-taking, since support people are too busy at this time; also discuss such plans with your birth center or hospital staff.

• Have your bag ready for an easy, relaxed departure (see the checklist below).

+

WHAT TO PACK

For Yourself

☐ 2 short nightgowns or shirts

☐ 1 bathrobe

☐ 1 change of underwear

☐ 1 pair of socks

☐ 1 pair of slippers

☐ 1 belt for feminine napkins

Your regular toilet articles, including:

☐ toothbrush and toothpaste

☐ comb and brush

☐ deodorant

☐ other items such as lip balm, hair ribbon, etc.

Items advised by the birth center or hospital, such as:

☐ shampoo

☐ shower cap

☐ washcloth and towel

☐ soap in a container

☐ plastic squeeze bottle for perineal care after birth

For Your Support Person:

Any items advised by the birth center or hospital, such as:

☐ 1 pair washable slippers or rubber thong sandals

☐ 1 T-shirt and shorts (or slacks), or warm-up suit (that is, casual, comfortable clothes for hot, hard work while helping)

☐ toilet articles

☐ washcloth and towel

For Your Baby
(Launder all baby clothes before using)

☐ 2 undershirts

☐ several diapers (disposable ones are usually provided by the birth center or hospital)

☐ 3 receiving blankets

☐ comb and brush

☐ if weather is cool, an outdoor outfit (with a hat) and a blanket or shawl to wrap the baby

Food and Beverages (If Allowed)

☐ nourishment for you during labor, such as:

fruit juices	ginger ale
soups	ice cream
yogurt	lollipops
tea	frozen fruit-juice cubes
honey for tea	jello

☐ easily prepared foods for support person (and your child or children with baby-sitter) such as fruit, sandwiches, juice, ice cream

☐ sturdy disposable cups, plates, napkins, and flatware

Optional Items (Or As You're Advised)

☐ things to keep you occupied and cheerful; books, games, tapes or radio, small TV, plants, flowers, a favorite small picture

☐ things to keep your child(ren) occupied, such as toys, games, books, dolls

☐ if you like, special foods and drinks to celebrate the birth (birth centers usually have a kitchen where families can prepare foods; check to see if such an option is available if you plan a hospital birth)

If the Baby Is Not in a Head-Down Position

Most likely, your baby will settle into the head-down position shown in Figure 13.1. This is the position babies take in more than 95 out of every 100 pregnancies. But in about 3 of every 100 cases, the baby settles with buttocks down and head up—in a breech presentation. And in the few remaining cases the baby takes some other unusual position.

Your care-giver will be able to tell by gentle palpation during your checkup visits what position the baby is in. You and your support partner may learn how to do this too in your prenatal classes, since it's not difficult.

"External version" may be suggested by your care-giver if your baby is still not head-down when you're within three or four weeks of the due date; not all professionals agree it should be attempted. Changing the baby's position should be done only by a trained, experienced professional. The professional manipulates the fetus from the outside while you're lying on your back, to get it to turn gradually into the head-down position.

If the baby remains in a position other than head-down as you advance to within a few days of your labor, talk with your care-giver about decisions to be made for labor and birth. Some professionals will go right ahead with the normal course of labor and a vaginal delivery in the case of babies in the breech presentation. The type of breech will be a factor in decision-making. Others advise cesarean section births for all breech or unusual presentations. (This is one of the questions we have suggested you ask potential care-providers.)

When You Go Beyond the Due Date

As you approach your due date, remember that it is only an approximation, a best guess. In normal births with spontaneous labors, about 30 out of every 100 babies arrive *before* their due dates—in a few of those 30 instances, even two weeks or more before the date.

Late arrivals are more than twice as common. Some 65 out of 100 arrive *after* their due dates—with about 10 out of every 100 coming more than ten days beyond their date.

You might wait longer than two weeks after your due date without being concerned, if your care-giver sees no problem. Some women having a first baby go as long as eighteen days or more past the due date and then have normal spontaneous labors and healthy babies.

A main concern of your care-giver will be the functioning of the placenta, should your pregnancy continue two weeks or more past the due date. With pregnancies that go beyond forty weeks, the placenta may become less able to transfer nutrients to the fetus. As a result, the unborn baby may be deprived to a point at which its health and even life are at risk. Before this point is reached, care-givers will try to ascertain how the baby is faring and may advise inducing labor or birth by a cesarean section.

Various tests indicate whether the baby is showing "fetal distress" and is endangered. One consists of a twenty-four-hour urine test; another is a blood test that is repeated on successive days. Others include a nonstress test (NST) and an oxytocin challenge test (OCT), both using electronic fetal monitoring, as described in Chapter 6. Some obstetricians advise weekly stress tests as a precaution after a pregnancy's forty-second week.

Another informative test is one you can do yourself. It is a simple matter of observation and recording. A physically active fetus is a strong, well-nourished one. At least ten strong movements in a twelve-hour period usually indicates that the baby is healthy.

Find a convenient time of day when you can focus on the baby's movements. Try to do the test at the same time every day. Note the time, then start counting the baby's movements until you reach ten and make a note of the finishing time. This should happen in a comparatively brief period of time, perhaps three to four hours or even less. Babies vary in their activity just as do adults. If you note fewer than ten in a twelve-hour period, contact your care-provider.

Call your care-giver if the baby's pattern of movements changes substantially. *Call immediately if you notice a cessation of movements or none in a six-hour period.*

How and When Labor Might Be Induced

Almost all expectant women whose condition and prenatal preparation clearly indicate normal, low-risk births go into labor spontaneously—without needing to have labor induced. In rare instances women and their partners, on their care-giver's advice, may decide that it's wise to have labor induced.

This possibility might result from either of two situations around (or after) the due date:

- Labor does not follow the breaking of the amniotic sac ("rupture of the membranes") and loss of amniotic fluid within a number of hours, usually twenty-four. (Birth centers tend to use a shorter twelve-hour time period when this occurs anytime between three or less weeks before and two weeks after the due date.

• Definite evidence of fetal distress, as indicated by counting fetal movements, by other observations such as fetal heart rate, or by tests such as NSTs or OCTs.

Ask your care-giver to explain the alternatives, with the reasons for and against each course of action, if this should happen to develop in your case.

If at any time your membranes break, inform your care-giver *immediately*. Your care-giver would be concerned mainly with the possibility of the cord prolapsing or of infection of the fetus or yourself.

It is likely that you will be asked to visit your provider for:

1. A check of your vital signs including temperature;

2. A test of your vaginal discharge to see if nitrazine paper confirms that the leaking is, in fact, amniotic fluid;

3. An examination with only a sterile speculum introduced into the vagina in order to check for the presence of the umbilical cord;

4. A careful check of the fetal heart rate. If cord is seen or the heart rate indicates distress a cesarean section would be performed. If all seems well the alternatives would be:

   • Wait to see if labor starts spontaneously, while taking steps to avoid and watch carefully for signs of infection. How long to wait is a matter of opinion, for some care-providers it is no longer than twenty-four hours; others will wait longer. During this time nothing is introduced into the vagina and your temperature is monitored in order to detect any possibility of infection.

   • Induce labor (chiefly to avoid risk of infection) if your cervix should be ready to respond to induction.

   • Deliver the baby by cesarean section if infection is threatening and if your cervix is not ready to dilate in response to induction.

To protect against and watch for possible signs of infection, your care-giver would probably advise no swimming, no tub baths (showers or sponge baths instead), no intercourse, no tampons, and no manual vaginal examinations. You would be asked to take your temperature every morning and night and report immediately if it's more than about one-half degree above the normal 98.6°. If conditions seem to warrant, you would be given blood tests every other day (or every day) to determine the white blood count. (A higher than normal count indicates infection.)

Actions like these are usually followed by labor starting spontaneously and proceeding normally. Do not be concerned about tales of "dry birth" you may have heard. There really is no such thing.

If your care-giver grows increasingly concerned about possible infection and is of the impression that your cervix is sufficiently softened and thinned to make induction feasible, he or she will secure your consent to do so.

In the second instance, that of fetal distress, it is likely that a cesarean section will be the appropriate means of managing the situation, particularly if the distress is marked by a much lowered fetal heart rate and the presence of meconium or if the cord has prolapsed.

One key consideration in decision-making regarding ruptured membranes is the vaginal examination which is usually required to determine cervical condition; it increases the risk of infection and thus should not be done without a convincing reason. Another factor is the condition of your cervix. An attempt to induce labor will probably fail unless your cervix is sufficiently softened by hormonal action and sufficiently thinned by Braxton-Hicks contractions. Specifically, it should have changed from being tightly closed to having opened about the diameter of one finger (2 centimeters). Labor can seldom be induced successfully unless such changes have started naturally.

If you and your care-giver decide to try to induce labor, you will be admitted to the hospital. In a labor room there, you will be given small quantities of dilute oxytocin by intravenous drip. Oxytocin is a hormone that stimulates the uterus to contract, as noted in Chapter 6. Care-givers often refer to it by one of the trade names under which it is marketed, such as Pitocin or Syntocinon. Properly administered IV oxytocin should gradually start strong labor contractions, which will continue until your baby is born vaginally.

You will also have electronic fetal monitoring if your labor is induced or stimulated with an oxytocin IV. Contractions can become extremely strong with oxytocin, and monitoring is needed in order to be sure that these strong contractions do not result in fetal distress.

If signs of infection appear and if your cervix is not ready, your care-giver will probably advise a cesarean section.

When Labor Should *Not* be Induced

Aside from its use in rupture of the membranes, you should consider deciding against having labor induced under these conditions:

• When the major reason is to have labor occur at a convenient time for either your care-giver or yourself. Such elective induction of labor became common in past decades. Virtually all childbearing authorities today advise against it.

This practice frequently led to the need for cesarean deliveries because the induction often failed to result in a "normal" labor. Needless premature births, respiratory problems in the infant after birth, and increased jaundice also resulted. In 1978 the U.S. Food and Drug Administration accordingly restricted its approval of oxytocin to its use in the elective induction of labor for the health and safety of mother and fetus only.[1]

- When examination shows that your cervix has not softened, thinned out, and begun dilating sufficiently to ensure continuation of labor if it is artificially induced.

- When oxytocin is administered in a way that its absorption by your system can't be carefully controlled, such as by subcutaneous injection.

The Stages of Labor

Advance Signs of Labor

You'll probably have been feeling what are often described as "rehearsal" contractions of your uterus at irregular times for a number of weeks. These Braxton-Hicks contractions are likely to have made your uterine muscles tighten noticeably. They probably also continued in no regular, rhythmic pattern. They usually become noticeable at some point after the fourth or fifth month of pregnancy and are part of the physiology of the expansion of the uterus. You may confuse them with the baby's movements. A hand on the abdomen will confirm overall tightening.

Here are some basic signs by which you might recognize the warm-up contractions of "false labor":

- False labor contractions tend to feel strong when you're lying down but weaker when you get up and walk around, take a shower, or are similarly active. However, in infrequent cases the reverse might be true.

- False labor contractions occur at irregular intervals and don't steadily increase in intensity.

- False labor contractions make your abdomen and uterus tighten up for a couple of minutes or more (in contrast to the half-minute or slightly more of early labor contractions).

Should the contractions continue and should you feel uncertain about them, report what's going on to your childbearing care-giver. It can sometimes be very hard to tell the difference between false and true labor contractions. The test is whether on pelvic examination your care-giver finds that your cervix is being effaced and dilated.

When Labor Starts

Specific physical developments take place with the start of actual labor, but the time at which they occur can vary widely from one woman to another.

- *Show:* A vaginal discharge of clear mucus tinged with blood. It appears after the mucus plug that has sealed the cervix is loosened by the contractions. It may occur at any time between several days before labor and some hours after labor has begun.

- *Rupture of the membranes:* A flow of clear fluid from the vagina— from a trickle to several cupfuls or more. This occurs when the amniotic sac breaks spontaneously. This too can happen anytime: before labor begins or several hours along in labor. *Always inform your care-giver if there is any possibility you are leaking amniotic fluid.*

- *Regular contractions that gradually increase in strength:* Labor contractions are stronger or more intense than warm-up contractions. You can recognize this by the increased tightening or tensing of your abdomen with each contraction. There is no lessening in intensity when you walk around or have a warm shower. You will feel a steady rise in the intensity and length of the contractions. (Remember that you may sense contractions as backache, indigestion, menstrual-like cramps, or bowel cramps. A hand on the abdomen will help you know if these sensations are, in fact, contractions.)

  Contractions will be lasting 20 or 30 seconds and with intervals between contractions lasting 10 or 8 minutes at the outset. However, there may be irregularity for several hours, and sometimes for the entire labor.

  Contractions will continue for 2 hours or more in one pattern of length and frequency, or with each contraction lasting longer and the intervals becoming shorter.

Tell your care-giver as soon as show or amniotic fluid flow occurs. Should you see either of the first two signs before strong and regular labor contractions have begun, call your care-giver right away. Either one can happen quite normally some time before labor, but you should report either or both should they occur. It's wise to see if there is any need for you to be examined or observed.

When regular contractions develop, phone your care-giver and discuss whether or not you're in labor. Be prepared to answer these questions:

- Has amniotic fluid started flowing? If so, when? Light or heavy? What color is it? Is there an odor?

- Is there a mucus discharge? Started when? What color? What consistency? Is it bloody? Is there a flow? Would you describe it as spotting? Would you describe it as bleeding?

- Describe your contractions: When did they start? How intense? How long do they last? How long are the intervals? Where do you feel them? Is it necessary to use your breathing techniques to ease them? If you are in labor, your care-giver should tell you when to arrive at the birth center or hospital, when he or she will arrive there, and anything you and/or your support person should be doing in the time being.

What sometimes seems to be false labor may be a relatively longer starting stage of actual labor, called prodromal labor. Such long-drawn-out initial labor can be very strong. It can also prove very tiring and discouraging because the cervix is being thinned and opened much more slowly than usually. Should you develop prodromal labor, follow your care-giver's suggestions, rest as much as possible, and keep up your nutritional intake.

What to Do if You Start Having the Baby Early

What if you should start delivering the baby while on the way, or even before you leave home (or at home before your care-provider arrives)? First, you should realize that this almost never happens with first labors. Moreover, "emergency" (or professionally unattended) childbirth is usually discussed in prenatal classes.

If you think you're starting to deliver the baby before you leave home, make yourself comfortable near the phone, call your care-provider, and follow her or his advice. It has happened that nurse-midwives and physicians have assisted women and their support partners through birth by telephone. In cases like these, the care-givers usually explain what the mothers and support partners are seeing and what to do to help the birth along without interfering.

If you are on your way to the birth center or hospital and start delivering the baby, follow these guidelines:

1. Try blowing out in quick puffs with fast intakes of breath between, like a dog panting. This will keep you from pushing.
2. Should you still feel the baby moving on down and out anyway, stop holding back. Just let the baby be born.
3. When you have given birth, pick the baby up gently, with your little finger wipe out its mouth gently to clear any mucus, and then cover it with a coat, blouse, or blanket and hold it face down against your chest for warmth. Keep the baby's head a little lower than its body, to facilitate drainage of mucus before crying takes place.
4. Leave the umbilical cord hanging loose without being pinched or cut.
5. As soon as the baby has cried vigorously and is breathing well, put it to your breast and encourage sucking, if you can. This will facilitate separation of the placenta and prevent undue bleeding.
6. Proceed to a hospital or birth center as soon as you safely can.

Starting Teamwork with Your Support Partner

Tell your support partner right away when you think you're starting in labor, and describe what's going on. He or she should make arrangements to stay with you, providing companionship that is relaxed, calm, and confident. As part of the team, he or she will:

- Help you get some sleep if the contractions start during the night.
- See that you get tasty, easily digested, nutritious foods to eat frequently in small amounts.
- Keep up your fluid intake, even if you don't feel like eating.
- Keep you company if the contractions start during the day, and spend time with you talking, reading, walking around at home, or outdoors, watching TV, and playing table games or card games.
- Check on the preparations, seeing that a bag is packed for the birth center or hospital, or that any remaining household arrangements are made if a home birth is planned.
- Help you stay comfortable as the contractions continue and build in intensity: setting up a comfortable chair where you can sit with your head, back, arms, and legs supported; giving you a hand when you want to walk around; and helping you pause and relax through a contraction.
- Help you hold off on special breathing until the contractions get strong enough for you to need controlled breathing. Then, when

you do, guide and join with you in the "basic relaxation breathing" you've practiced together (see page 149).

• Help you time the contractions. For this, you or your partner should time several series of four or five contractions each. Let an hour or two pass between your timing of each series of contractions. Your aim is to be able to tell roughly how long each contraction lasts, and how many minutes there are on the average between contractions. This information will help you and your care-giver assess how your labor is progressing.

Your partner should try to be especially patient and understanding through any "false alarms." In the last two or three weeks of your pregnancy you might experience some very intense Braxton-Hicks contractions. You might think that labor is occurring at last and then be very disappointed when they quiet down and stop.

Remember that these warm-up contractions are a good workout for your uterus, and they should make for an easier, better labor and birth when the time is right.

Expect Early Labor to Go On for 6 to 12 Hours

Once your contractions are long enough and strong enough to show that labor has begun, check with your care-provider who will likely tell you to relax and keep occupied at home as your contractions lengthen, intensify, and gradually occur at closer intervals. Continue to time them and keep a record.

Your care-giver will tell you when to head for the birth center or hospital (if you're not having a home birth). This timing varies, depending on many factors—among them, how long a trip it is, how fast your labor seems to be going, and whether or not this is your first baby.

For some labors and some expectant parents, labor goes very quickly and the baby arrives just a few hours after labor seems to have started.

However, the early or latent phase of labor generally runs for 6 to 12 hours or more. Care-givers usually think you'll be more comfortable at home through the long hours of this beginning phase, so plan on managing as well as possible through it at home, whether or not you plan a home birth.

First-Stage Labor

You and your support partner can manage through labor and birth by knowing in detail what is happening in your body.

The essential, major development that takes place in first-stage labor is effacement and dilation of the cervix—its gradual stretching and opening, brought about by the successive waves of contractions in order to let the baby's head through. You might envision it by thinking of your uterus as a turtleneck sweater (Figure 13.1), which you're putting on the baby. You stretch the turtleneck so it will open and slide over the baby's head. The contractions of your uterus stretch your cervix over the baby's head.

The baby's head and body are moving deeper into your pelvis at the same time as your cervix is dilating in first-stage labor. This moving-down is called "descent."

Braxton-Hicks contractions in the days before labor start the process of softening up, thinning, and stretching the cervix.

The most common position for the baby as labor starts is the head-down, or "vertex," presentation; it occurs in about 95 percent of all pregnancies. And the specific head-down position—the "left occiput anterior" position—is the most common one in vertex presentations.

Various other anterior or posterior head-down positions of the fetus in early labor normally pose no special problems for the mother. During labor you may hear them referred to by your care-givers with acronyms such as "LOA" and "ROP" (left occiput anterior, and right occiput posterior).

However, in posterior positions, the head of the fetus can press against the mother's lower spine during labor. The head is also less effectively situated for helping to dilate the cervix. Labor with the fetus in a posterior position can therefore be long, slow, and difficult, particularly for a mother having her first baby.

Your care-giver can tell you if your baby is in a posterior position in early labor. He or she can also guide you and your support partner on using special techniques to cope with the resulting "back labor." Pressure on the mother's lower back by her support partner and care-givers can often prove especially helpful in such labor. The techniques include use of ice or heat, and positioning of the woman's body.

During labor you may hear your care-givers use the term "station" as well as "position." Station refers to descent and is a description of the progress of the baby through the mother's pelvis. Engagement (page 197) is station zero. If the baby's head (or breech) has not reached the level of the ischial spines, it is said to be at a minus station (−1 or −2). As the baby's head passes the ischial spines it is said to be at a plus station (+1, +2). Plus three is the equivalent of being seen at the vaginal opening.

IN LABOR: UTERUS IS CONTRACTING,
CERVIX DILATING, BAG OF WATERS BELOW HEAD

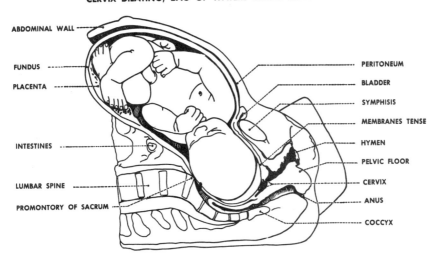

ABDOMINAL WALL

FUNDUS

PLACENTA

INTESTINES

LUMBAR SPINE

PROMONTORY OF SACRUM

PERITONEUM

BLADDER

SYMPHISIS

MEMBRANES TENSE

HYMEN

PELVIC FLOOR

CERVIX

ANUS

COCCYX

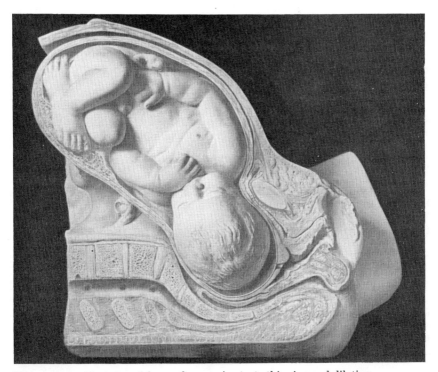

Figure 13.2. First-stage labor—after cervix starts thinning and dilating

215

Dilation of the cervix progresses gradually, along with other important changes such as descent and rotation of the baby's head.*

You can expect to dilate from 2 to 10 centimeters during first-stage labor. Midwives and obstetricians use centimeter measurements formally, but during labor they may refer to "finger" measurements to indicate the amount of cervical opening. Dilation is determined at various times during labor by tracing gently around the edge of the cervical opening with a gloved finger and estimating the diameter in numbers of finger-widths. One finger is the equivalent of 2 centimeters, and 5 fingers represents full dilation, about 10 centimeters. Early first stage is referred to as the latent phase. In this period of 6–8 hours on average effacement and dilation up to 3 centimeters takes place. The first stage is said then to go into an active phase lasting perhaps 3–5 hours during which dilation progresses from 3–8 centimeters. The final 1–2 hours of first-stage labor are referred to as transition.

What happens and how to cope with it as you and your support partner progress through first-stage labor are summarized in the following guide. This outlines what happens in a typical labor with a first-born child. Individual labors differ widely, however. Be ready to adapt to developments that may depart from the typical pattern.

The actions described are ones you would typically utilize in a family-centered labor at a birth center or hospital, or at home. The different ways in which your labor and birth experience would probably be managed if you are having a conventional hospital birth are described at the end of the chapter.

During first-stage labor, your professional care-giver will periodically check your blood pressure, pulse, temperature, and respiration, and the baby's heartbeat with a stethoscope or a similar instrument, a fetoscope. You will also be given vaginal examinations to check the progress of labor.

Expect your labor contractions to intensify gradually with the passing hours of first-stage labor. Relying more and more on teamwork with your partner and using techniques you've learned can help you manage as you move into the active phase of the first stage of labor.

---

* Rotation is another aspect of normal labor. It refers to the turning of the baby to accommodate the smallest diameter of the presenting part to the planes of the mother's pelvis. Figure 13.4 shows the way the fetus' head turns from an oblique position facing the mother's side to a face-down position (occiput anterior) for actual birth. Posterior babies must rotate farther or be born looking up (occiput posterior) which is referred to as a "sunny side up" birth.

Guide for Early First-Stage Labor

Physical Developments

Cervix is effacing and dilating up to 3 centimeters. (Figure 13.2B)

Initial contractions become regular, lasting about 30 to 50 seconds, and coming at intervals of 10, 8, and then 6 or so minutes apart. Starting contractions are mild, somewhat like strong menstrual cramps.

Possible backache in lower back.

Possible discomfort in lower abdomen and a sense of pelvic pressure.

Bloody show may appear.

Amniotic membranes may break, with release of amniotic fluid.

Contractions gradually building in intensity and length.

Your Feelings

Excitement and relief that labor has really begun.

Some anxious wondering about what's ahead, and impulses to talk and socialize.

Actions for You and Your Partner

Reassure yourselves that you are doing fine.

Move around, be active at home; perhaps go out for a walk or a movie.

Have one or more light meals for energy.

Urinate every hour.

Do pelvic rock exercises to counteract backache and relieve other discomfort.

Use relaxation exercises—whole-body relaxation and breathing, partial-body relaxation, and touch relaxation with your partner.

Use relaxation breathing—slow, deep, even breathing—once you feel the need to.

If the amniotic sac breaks, see if the fluid is clear. *Report this development to your care-giver.*

For Your Partner Especially

Press against her lower back with the heel of the hand (possibly hard, if she wants) to relieve backache.

Use touch relaxation techniques on muscles she's tensing, as you've practiced together. Help her to remain generally relaxed.

Once she starts controlled breathing, help her carry out relaxation breathing through each contraction; do the breathing with her on some contractions as they get stronger.

Time her contractions.

GUIDE FOR ACTIVE FIRST-STAGE LABOR

Physical Developments

Cervix is dilating from about 3 centimeters to about 8 centimeters.

Contractions grow stronger and run up to a full minute in length with only 5 to 3 minutes between.

Your Feelings

Increasing urge to stay quiet, to go into deep concentration for each contraction without talking or moving.

Increased need to have trusted persons nearby.

At times, doubts about your ability to do it, and difficulty in seeing an end to the process.

Actions for You and Your Partner

Try to make sure your surroundings are quiet and peaceful.

During contractions, sit up or lie on your side, or get on hands and knees if your back aches, and use slow deep breathing.

Change positions and move around as you may need in order to feel more comfortable.

Remember to use a deep cleansing breath before and especially after your rhythmic deep breathing through each contraction (to keep the baby well supplied with oxygen).

Have some light food and liquids between contractions (such as Jell-O, toast, juice, and honey-flavored tea).

Urinate every hour to keep your bladder empty.

Don't think ahead; just stay calm through the present moment.

If needed, use modified shallow breathing, but only at the peak of a contraction.

For Your Partner Especially

Give her frequent, quiet reassurance by saying things like "You're doing fine," "Keep it up," and general praise. Positive observations can also help, such as, "The contraction is at its peak, it'll be easing off soon."

Keep the surroundings calm and relaxing, without glaring lights, noisy activity, and needless talking.

Slow her down and help her deepen her breathing if she starts to use shallow breathing too early. Later join her in shallow breathing if she needs it at the peak of a contraction.

For backache, apply firm pressure to her lower back; having her take a hands-and-knees position may help; a heating pad, hot shower, or ice packs may bring relief, too.

For fluids, she may welcome cold juice, cracked ice, or ice chips (particularly ones made with fruit juice).

Thoughtful actions can be very comforting, like mopping her face and neck with a cool, damp cloth, applying chapstick to her dry lips, propping her up with pillows, gentle effleurage on the abdomen, helping her shift position and move around, or giving her gentle hugs.

Help her focus only on the present contraction and not think ahead.

As labor becomes highly intense, take a break from the strenuous work of support while a care-giver relieves you. Eat some food and relax a bit.

As advised by your care-giver, you will probably be at (or on your way to) the birth center or hospital in this phase (or attended by your care-giver if you're having a home birth).

You'll reach full dilation as first-stage labor ends. At half dilation, your condition will be essentially as pictured in Figure 13.2A. Note in particular on the labeled diagram how the cervix has opened over the top of the baby's head. The part labeled "external os anterior"

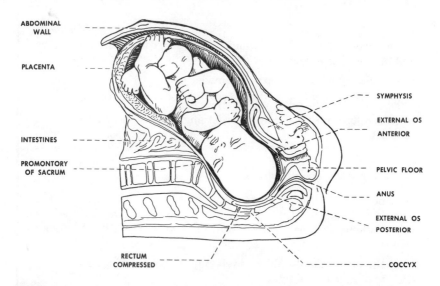

ABDOMINAL WALL

PLACENTA

INTESTINES

PROMONTORY OF SACRUM

SYMPHYSIS

EXTERNAL OS ANTERIOR

PELVIC FLOOR

ANUS

EXTERNAL OS POSTERIOR

RECTUM COMPRESSED

COCCYX

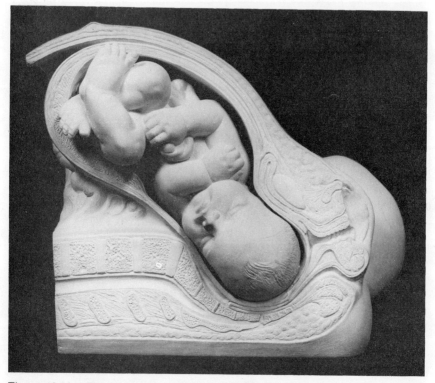

Figure 13.2A. First-stage labor midway—half dilation of cervix

indicates the front edge of the cervical opening, and "external os posterior" indicates the rear edge of the opening. (In the illustration, the membranes have not ruptured. This is the case in many labors.)

Transition to Second-Stage Labor

Nearly full dilation will bring you to what many women find the most difficult phase of labor, "transition." This phase closes first-stage labor and leads to second-stage labor, which culminates in the baby's birth.

Concentrate on your coping techniques through transition, rather than giving thought to how hard it may be. Doing so has helped many expectant women manage without panic and with little or no pain-killing medication on through transition and birth.

Shortly before or in transition, you and your care-giver may decide that you would be helped if given a mild dose of pain-killing medication. One medication commonly given is an injection of meperidene (Demerol). But there is no need to have medication if you don't want it or feel it necessary.

GUIDE FOR TRANSITION PHASE

Physical Developments

Contractions come only 3 to 1½ minutes apart, seeming to be one right after the other.

Contractions become intense almost immediately after they begin, and remain intense almost the entire time; they last for a full minute or more (60 to 90 seconds).

Possible nausea, sometimes accompanied by vomiting.

Shaking and cramps in your legs.

Increased bloody show and fluid discharge. If the amniotic sac hasn't broken yet, it is likely to do so at this point.

Heavy perspiration, but your feet may be cold.

Your Feelings

Irritable and sensitive to the slightest annoyance; you may not even want to be touched.

Contractions seem to give you no respite.

Panicky feelings at seeing no way out.

Nervous, tense; find it very hard to relax.

Annoyed by any clothing you have on; relief after taking it off.

Possible strong urge to have a bowel movement, or push, as transition ends and second-stage labor starts. This is caused by the pressure of the baby's head on the rectum.

Actions for You and Your Partner

Assume whatever position feels most comfortable for you; lying on one side is often preferred, though some women find relief in sitting, squatting, or getting on hands and knees.

Use shallow breathing through the long peaks of the contractions; take extra cleansing breaths after (and before) contractions to supply oxygen to the baby.

Blow out in puffs as needed to keep from pushing or bearing down.

For Your Partner Especially

Stay with her and don't leave for a second during transition. (Take a break beforehand.)

Talk to her and keep eye contact with her through every contraction; guide her through the pattern of extra cleansing breaths and shallow breathing, often breathing along with her.

Don't let her worry about what's ahead; have her focus on this one contraction, at this instant.

If she's gripped by momentary panic and confusion while in a contraction, say in a firm voice, "Breathe in, breathe out, keep it up, keep it even," and so on through the contraction.

If she's been given medication, she may doze off between contractions and wake confused; if so, as the contraction starts tell her firmly to keep her eyes open and follow the breathing reminders.

Give her sips of fluid to drink, or ice chips for her dry mouth.

Dry her face with a cloth; cool her face with a dampened cloth.

If she feels like pushing, urge her to blow out in intermittent puffs to keep from pushing, at least until examined by her care-giver.

Perhaps give gentle rhythmic massage on the insides of her thighs, if it gives relief.

Possibly apply pressure to her lower back if she has backache.

If she has a very strong urge to push, tell her it's all right to push gently (unless the care-giver says no).

If she says she has an urge to move her bowels, report this to the care-giver (it may signal the start of second-stage labor).

Hold on if you can without panicking through transition, especially by working to get through it moment by moment. It's a relatively short period in most cases, lasting only an hour or two. Each contraction brings you one step closer to having your baby. And it's followed by what usually feels like enormous relief in second-stage labor—when hard work will culminate in birth.

Second-Stage Labor

The second stage covers the period of time from full dilatation of the cervix to the actual birth, one to two hours. During this stage you will work to move the baby from your body into the outer world.

GUIDE FOR SECOND-STAGE LABOR

Physical Developments

Contractions come farther apart, letting you rest and gather strength between.

Contractions continue strong and run about 60 to 100 seconds in length.

Baby starts moving down through the opened cervix into the birth canal.

Contractions cause urge to push or bear down to help in moving the baby down and out.

Your Feelings

Welcome relief and excitement at first, with renewed ability to talk and be social.

Possible interludes of discouragement as labor seems to keep going on and on and the baby still isn't born.

Possible lack of urge to push, or fear that pushing will hurt you.

Actions for You and Your Partner

Push only when you feel a very strong urge to do so. Don't push if there is only a slight urge, even though you may be impatient to push.

Take two deep cleansing breaths as you feel each contraction starting; these help provide vital oxygen to the baby.

Assume a position squatting, on hands and knees, lying on your side, or sitting propped up—whichever feels best to you for contractions and pushing.

Use your second-stage breathing exercises, as practiced with your partner (see page 158).

Use your "pushing breathing" (pages 158, 160) when you're ready.

For Your Partner Especially

Keep praising her for how well she is doing.

Help guide her through proper breathing, pushing, and not pushing, as her care-giver advises.

Help her relax her jaw, shoulders, legs, and pelvic floor especially, perhaps by using touch relaxation.

Encourage her not to feel impatient or rushed; remind her that her pelvic muscles and tissues need to be stretched out gradually, and that this takes time (particularly for a first child).

What happens at this time in second-stage labor is portrayed in Figure 13.3. Illustrated there is a fairly unusual condition in which the amniotic sac has not yet broken. The cervical edges have pulled up and well along over the baby's head, as reflected by the parts labeled "external os."

224

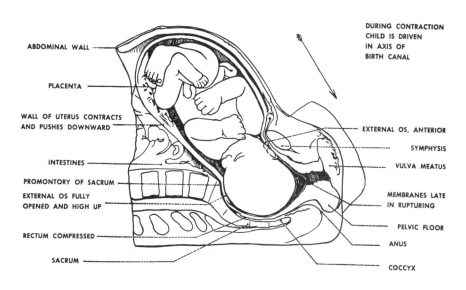

ABDOMINAL WALL

PLACENTA

WALL OF UTERUS CONTRACTS
AND PUSHES DOWNWARD

INTESTINES

PROMONTORY OF SACRUM

EXTERNAL OS FULLY
OPENED AND HIGH UP

RECTUM COMPRESSED

SACRUM

DURING CONTRACTION
CHILD IS DRIVEN
IN AXIS OF
BIRTH CANAL

EXTERNAL OS, ANTERIOR

SYMPHYSIS

VULVA MEATUS

MEMBRANES LATE
IN RUPTURING

PELVIC FLOOR

ANUS

COCCYX

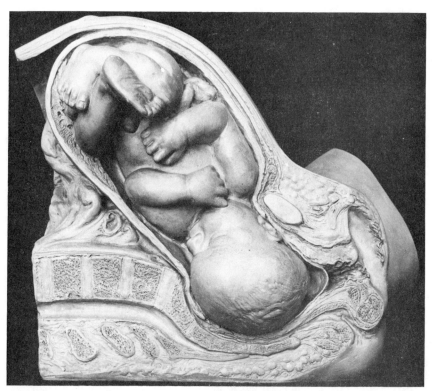

Figure 13.3.   Second-stage labor—baby moving through birth canal

Birth

Birth itself comes not long after, as the culminating and concluding phase of second-stage labor.

<u>**GUIDE FOR BIRTH**</u>

Physical Developments

Contractions continue strong, running 60 to 90 seconds long and 2 or 3 minutes apart.

Urge to push intensifies with contractions.

Stretching of the skin of the pelvic floor as the baby's head "crowns," or pushes against it, to stretch it open and pass through. You will feel a burning sensation with this stretching, which makes you hold back and counteract the urge to push. This protects the pelvic floor tissues from tearing.

Your Feelings

Very powerful urges to bear down.

May feel confused, physically driven, and in special need of guidance by care-giver and partner in order to keep in contact with what's happening.

Desire to touch and see the baby as you're told the head is crowning and then emerging. (You can put a hand down to touch it and can be given a mirror to see it, when the time comes.)

More urges to bear down after the baby's head emerges.

Sharp sense of wondering if the baby's all right as soon as it's fully born. Then excitement, exhilaration, and disbelief that the baby is really born. Sometimes you become tearful in the midst of your happiness.

Actions for You and Your Partner

Keep up the second-stage breathing, using "do push" and "do not push" sequences as your care-giver advises. (Your care-giver may also be mas-

---

saging your perineum and holding the baby's head gently to help the perineum stretch.)

Listen carefully to what your care-giver advises.

Stop pushing, by panting or blowing, when you feel the burning sensation of your pelvic floor stretching.

When your care-giver says the baby's head is crowning, stop pushing when the care-giver suggests, and hold your mouth open with light-chest breathing (or panting) as the baby's head eases out.

For Your Partner Especially

Reassure her that she really does have herself under control and is doing just fine.

Talk quietly to her all the time with praise and encouragement.

Offer sips of liquid in between contractions, and a cool cloth for her forehead.

Remind her to listen closely to her care-giver's directions, and to stop pushing when she feels the burning sensations in her pelvic floor.

Join the care-giver in urging her to reach down and help in the final stage of birth.

Share in the excitement and wonder with her as the baby is born.

How birth itself typically unfolds at the end of second-stage labor is portrayed in Figures 13.4, 13.5, and 13.6. Figure 13.4 shows how the baby's head "crowns," when its top can be seen emerging through the outlet of the vagina. Then in Figure 13.5, the emergence of the baby's entire head is illustrated. Finally, Figure 13.6 depicts how birth of the entire body is facilitated after the baby's shoulders and body have turned. After the baby's shoulders are born, the rest of the body slips out easily, with the care-giver gently supporting and guiding the baby's emergence.

Your attention, and your partner's, will understandably be focused on your new baby in these moments. The baby will be given to you to look over, cuddle, keep warm, and put to the breast either right away or in a short time (after having had breathing passages cleared and been given a quick assessment by your care-giver). Caring for and welcoming your baby starting with these very first moments of life is a subject we discuss in the next chapter.

Third-Stage Labor

While you're greeting the baby, you will also be going through the third and last stage of labor. This takes only minimum attention and effort on the part of yourself and your partner, and ends after you expel the placenta.

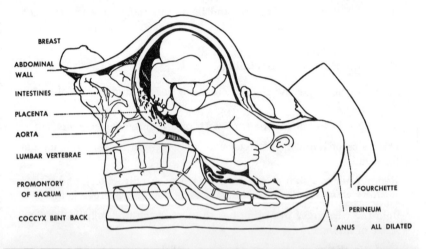

BREAST
ABDOMINAL WALL
INTESTINES
PLACENTA
AORTA
LUMBAR VERTEBRAE
PROMONTORY OF SACRUM
COCCYX BENT BACK
FOURCHETTE
PERINEUM
ANUS   ALL DILATED

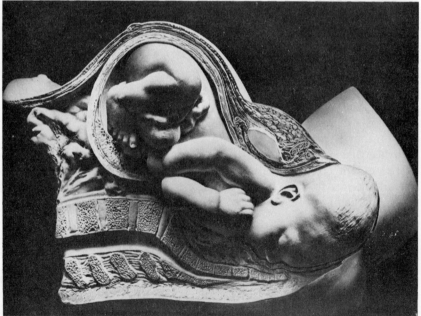

Figure 13.4. Second-stage labor—baby's head "crowns"

Contractions often stop temporarily after the baby's birth and then resume, but they are relatively painless. Contractions and shrinking of the uterus cause the placenta to separate from the uterine wall. You may feel an urge to push and may be asked to do so during the contractions.

After a few contractions the placenta is usually expelled, perhaps with the gentle assistance of the care-giver. The uterus then rises to

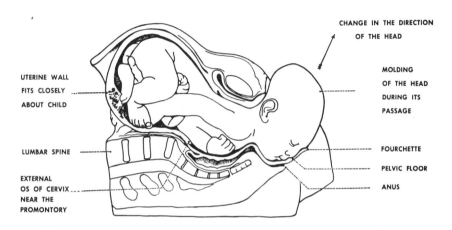

CHANGE IN THE DIRECTION
OF THE HEAD

MOLDING
OF THE HEAD
DURING ITS
PASSAGE

UTERINE WALL
FITS CLOSELY
ABOUT CHILD

LUMBAR SPINE

FOURCHETTE

PELVIC FLOOR

EXTERNAL
OS OF CERVIX
NEAR THE
PROMONTORY

ANUS

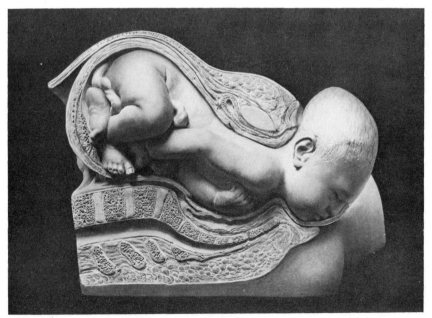

Figure 13.5. Second-stage labor ending—baby's head almost born

229

resume much the same position it had at about the sixteenth week of pregnancy (see Figures 13.7 and 13.8).

What to Expect with Conventional Hospital Management of Normal Labor and Birth

Your own and your partner's active participation may be curtailed if you are having a conventional hospital birth. The preceding guides outline actions through a family-centered normal labor in a hospital

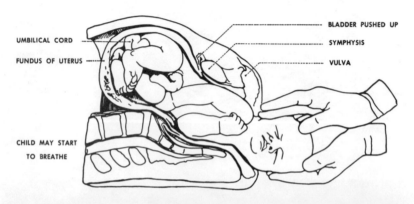

UMBILICAL CORD

FUNDUS OF UTERUS

CHILD MAY START
TO BREATHE

BLADDER PUSHED UP

SYMPHYSIS

VULVA

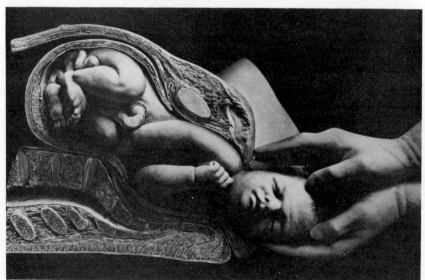

Figure 13.6. Second-stage labor—birth

or out-of-hospital birth center, or at home, but can be applied in some hospitals also.

The physical developments and your feelings will be the same in a conventional hospital birth up to the point at which you might receive anesthesia, particularly the epidural. After that you would have

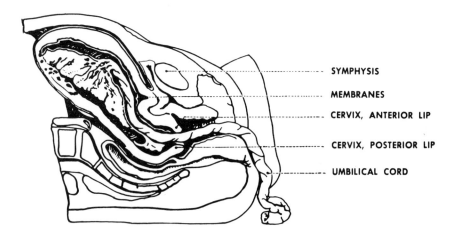

- - - - SYMPHYSIS

- - - - MEMBRANES

- - - - CERVIX, ANTERIOR LIP

- - - - CERVIX, POSTERIOR LIP

- - - - UMBILICAL CORD

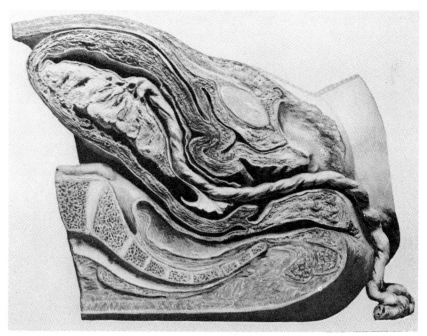

Figure 13.7. Third-stage labor—placenta separating from uterus wall

a dulled sensation of what was taking place in the lower part of your body. In addition, if permitted only at labor, your support partner might not be with you. You will be attended instead by the hospital nurses and your care-giver.

After being admitted to the hospital, you will go to the labor and delivery floor. Your support partner can usually stay in the room with you. At times, he or she may be asked to leave for a short period.

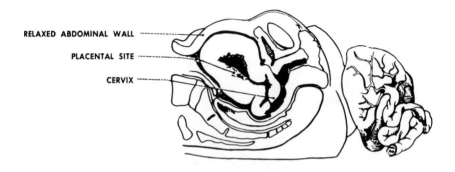

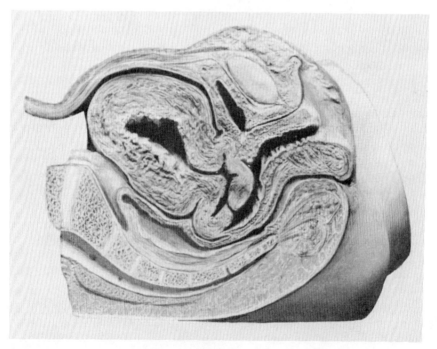

Figure 13.8. Third-stage labor—uterus after placenta is expelled

You might be given a partial or complete shave of your pubic hair, and an enema.

You might be connected to an external or internal electronic fetal monitor (EFM), which records your contractions and the fetal heart rate. Internal monitoring would require rupture of the amniotic membranes if they haven't already broken and you would have limited freedom to move. Having external monitoring is much like undergoing the contraction stress test described in Chapter 6. With internal monitoring, the condition of the fetus is recorded by attaching an electrode to the fetal scalp. A catheter into the uterus records the contractions. In external monitoring all recording is based on impulses which are detected through the abdominal wall. You may be disconnected from the monitor for short periods in order to walk around and go to the bathroom, provided you are on an external monitor.

Even though you have an EFM, you should ask to lie on your side. Do not lie on your back continuously because undue pressure is put on your circulatory system.

An intravenous feeding of a glucose solution will probably be started to keep you hydrated and to provide energy (since food and fluids by mouth are usually not allowed), and for convenience should you later need to have medication, such as oxytocin.

You might be taken to a labor room near the delivery room if you were not admitted there directly. You and your labor partner may be on your own there most of the time, except for periodic checks by the nurse or doctor.

As you move into the greater intensity of active first-stage contractions, you may be given a pain-killer like Demerol by injection or through the IV. If your contractions haven't produced full dilation after some hours, you may be given oxytocin via the IV to stimulate labor and make contractions more intense.

As you approach full dilation, you may be wheeled into the delivery room (similar to an operating room) and be asked to move onto the delivery table. Your legs will probably be placed in stirrups. You can ask for a backrest so you do not have to lie on your back. IV hookups will continue. You will be draped with sterile sheets and your perineal area will be cleansed with antiseptic.

If you did not have one earlier, an anesthesiologist may give you an epidural by injection in your lower back at about this time. You will be asked to sit up or lie on your side while this is done. With such regional anesthesia, you will have decreased ability to move the lower half of your body. Painful sensations will be greatly dulled, and your reflexes to push and your sensations of pelvic-floor stretching will also be substantially dulled.

In second-stage labor your care-giver will tell you when to push and when not to push.

At about the time the baby's head is crowning, you will probably be given an episiotomy after first receiving local anesthesia by injection (if you had not had an epidural). An episiotomy is an incision from the rear edge of the vaginal opening back toward the anal opening. It enlarges the vaginal opening for passage of the baby's head and shoulders. Sometimes the incision is made to one side.

Professional care-givers who practice traditional birth tend to think that episiotomies should be done in almost all deliveries, and especially in deliveries of women having their first child. Other practitioners try to avoid doing an episiotomy unless it appears absolutely necessary in order to avoid a jagged tear of the tissues. Factors like allowing more time for birth, from crowning on, and having good muscle tone in the pelvic floor (by doing Kegel exercises throughout pregnancy) appear to result in less frequent need for episiotomies. Prenatal perineal massage may also be helpful.

After being born your baby might be briefly shown to you and then taken off to the nursery. Or, if you plan to breastfeed, your baby might be given to you to nurse for a short time before being separated from you for an examination in the nursery. You would be moved to a recovery room where you will stay until the anesthetic wears off, and then to your maternity-floor room.

Your husband or any other waiting relatives or friends will be told by a nurse or the doctor of the baby's arrival and your condition. If you are not too tired, a couple of these persons at a time may visit you in your room (if the babies are not out of the nursery for a scheduled feeding with other mothers on the floor).

14

The New Family Member: Care, Bonding, and Feeding

In normal deliveries birth often ends quickly after the head and shoulders emerge. The baby's body naturally turns to permit the shoulders to pass through the largest diameter of the pelvis; then the baby comes out completely and easily with the next contraction.

Starting at that dramatic instant, here are the most important things for you, your partner, and your care-givers to do:

- With your loved ones take the time to enjoy that enormous sense of accomplishment and relief.

- Clear any mucus from the baby's nose and mouth frequently if necessary, for breathing. Your care-giver will do this after the head appears and while awaiting the completion of birth. This normally takes only a second or so. A soft rubber bulb is used to suction out mucus in the baby's nose and mouth so that the passageways are cleared.

- Welcome and "bond" with your new baby. You and your partner can gently cuddle, caress, and talk to him or her. The natural as well as the recommended way to do this is to hold the newborn so you and the baby can gaze directly into each other's eyes. Then touch and stroke your baby, first with your fingertips and then with your palms.

- Carry out some of the other aspects of a "gentle" birth (also known as the Leboyer approach to birth), such as avoiding overbright lights and loud noises, keeping voices low and soothing, and putting the baby against your skin for warmth.

- Confirm that your baby's all right. Your care-giver will assess the baby by doing an evaluation called an "Apgar score" at one minute and again at five minutes after the birth.
- Put your baby to your breast and let him or her start to suckle when ready (whether or not you plan to breastfeed; as explained before, this is for your benefit as well as the baby's).

Why Bonding with Your Baby Is Important

You and your newborn baby benefit by close physical contact right after birth, according to many child development professionals today. In their view, the newborn is comforted by immediate skin-to-skin contact. You can cuddle, caress, look at, and talk to your baby. The baby is given to you once the care-giver has checked to see that breathing is well established and everything is normal. You and the baby (to be sure its body temperature is maintained) will be covered with a blanket.

Having the father also hold his baby close, caress it, talk to it, and make eye contact is important for him and the baby too. Parental contact with the baby ideally should go on for at least twenty or thirty minutes, preferably without interruption.

Bonding not only satisfies spontaneous emotional responses of parents and their newborns but also facilitates normal physical and psychological development. Children welcomed this way right after birth have been found to have fewer subsequent health problems than other children. Analyses have also indicated that their parents interact with and enjoy them more than comparable parents who did not carry out such bonding.[1]

If you have the type of birth that doesn't allow bonding or a Leboyer approach, you can start bonding and attachment as soon as it is feasible for you and your baby. It is never "too late."

Gentle Birth

Many professionals today believe that newborns benefit from birth conditions that are gentle, quiet, softly lit, and peaceful. Bonding actions fit well with such a gentle birth approach.

You and your helpers should turn off any glaring, bright lights, talk softly, avoid loud noises of apparatus or utensils, and have the room comfortably warm. You should also handle the baby in a gentle, soothing way.

When received under conditions of gentle birth like these, newborn babies are often quiet and alert. They gaze with an intent expression into the eyes of anyone holding them. This peaceful, responsive behavior has led professionals to recommend a gentle birth environment rather than brightly lit settings of traditional hospital births. (Such conditions previously had been thought to be unimportant to newborns because they were too immature to sense anything.)

This gentle approach became more widely available even in hospital births after it was promoted by a French obstetrician Frederick Leboyer in his influential book *Birth Without Violence.* [2]

You and your partner (as well as the care-giver) may want to use an additional feature recommended by Dr. Leboyer—a bath for the baby. The newborn is immersed in warm water while the parent or care-giver supports it gently. This is especially soothing, according to Leboyer, because it is similar to the baby's experience of floating in the amniotic fluid before birth.

Newborn infants generally do seem comforted by such baths. Some couples prefer that the father give his baby the Leboyer bath while the mother watches and sometimes dips her hands in the water to massage and stroke the baby. Gentle stroking of the baby's body may be more important than actually bathing the baby in water.

Putting the Infant to the Breast to Nurse

In the early minutes after birth, you should offer your baby the opportunity to nurse. Some babies are not interested in doing so but will be more interested later. Nursing your baby is an integral part of bonding and gentle birth. If you plan to bottlefeed rather than breastfeed, you can still bond with your baby very effectively.

Letting your newborn breastfeed right after birth benefits you because nursing stimulates release of the body's natural oxytocin, which makes your uterus contract. Stimulating the uterus to contract after birth serves two purposes: It helps the uterus expel the placenta and decrease in size, and it helps prevent hemorrhaging after the birth by keeping the uterus firmly contracted.

Your baby benefits from being breastfed even for a short time starting at birth or soon after. As discussed earlier, your breasts initially secrete a sticky yellowish fluid called colostrum, which is a highly beneficial food for the newborn. It contains antibodies from your system that give your newborn important immunities. It is also high in protein and aids in excreting bilirubin (thereby helping to prevent jaundice in the newborn).

Moreover, nursing right after birth seems to be reassuring and comforting to newborn babies, as well as emotionally fulfilling to their mothers. Nursing also satisfies the newborn's intense need to suck. Infants will go on sucking long after their hunger is satisfied.

"Rooting"

At birth your newborn has a number of preprogrammed, or built-in, reflexes. These ensure breathing, crying, sucking, and swallowing, all essential activities for survival. Sneezing also helps keep breathing passages clear. Other inborn reflexes include:

- The "walking" or "stepping" reflex, in which the infant makes step-like movements with its legs if held upright; this reflex soon vanishes, and it does not reappear until the baby learns to walk a year or so later.
- The "grasp" reflex, in which its fingers tightly clamp on your finger.
- The "startle" reflex, in which a loud noise or rough handling causes the baby to tense its whole body with a jerk, flail its arms out as if to embrace something, and appear to shiver.
- "Rooting" for the nipple, in which the infant turns its head back and forth in seeking behavior; if touched on a cheek by a finger or a nipple, it will turn its head in that direction.

When you start to breastfeed you can take advantage of the rooting reflex to help your baby find the nipple. Sometimes it takes a few minutes or longer for the rooting reflex to appear. If your baby doesn't find and take the nipple right away, just be patient and let the baby rest its head against your breast from time to time. In a little while he or she probably will seek out the nipple and nurse. Some babies seem disinterested at first: this is not unusual.

If your care-giver is a midwife, she or he will assist you with breastfeeding. Or if you are in a hospital that permits immediate breastfeeding, the staff nurses will help you.

Your Baby's Health Care Right after Birth

For healthy newborns, getting to know you and your partner through bonding and sensing the world peacefully through gentle birth take precedence over routine health care that is performed after birth.

Cutting the Umbilical Cord

Even though obstetrical practice in past years included clamping and cutting the cord immediately after birth, there's no urgent reason to do so with a normal, healthy baby. Bonding between the parents and the baby first is now regarded as more important.

In numerous births today, at birth centers and hospitals as well as at home, it is the father who cuts the cord. Care-givers usually wait until the cord stops its pulsations, which can be seen or felt with the fingers. Then two small clamps are placed on the cord about 3 inches away from the baby's abdomen and about the width of a finger apart, and the cord is cut between the clamps with a pair of sterile surgical scissors. The baby feels nothing since there are no nerves in the cord.

The cord stump gradually dries, and after the fifth or sixth day it becomes blackened and falls off by itself. The final shape of the child's navel is not influenced in any way by how or when the cord was cut.

When the mother has had heavy labor medication, or if the baby has a low weight (under 5½ pounds), respiratory distress, or other health handicap, some precautions with the cord are usually taken. Before the cord is cut, these babies are kept at a lower level than the placenta—perhaps by being placed on the mother's thigh for first bonding. This attempts to ensure that all the baby's blood in the placenta will flow into its system (which can be as much as 10 to 15 percent of its initial blood supply).

The baby would not have the advantage of this additional blood were it placed higher than the placenta (say, on the mother's abdomen), since the placental blood cannot flow up to the baby after birth. Healthy babies manage well without the additional blood volume.

The First Things to Notice about Your Newborn Baby

You, your partner, and your care-giver will eagerly look over your baby right away. Here's what you're likely to see when all is well.

- *Crying and fast breathing:* At birth, healthy babies usually cry spontaneously as a way of inflating their lungs and starting to get their own oxygen from the air. How much and how loudly the baby cries—or how little and how softly—usually is just an individual difference. Babies also cough and gag, which helps them clear and spit up mucus in order to breathe. When they stop crying or doze off, their breathing rate is faster than your own.

- *Damp, soft skin:* The baby arrives still wet from the amniotic fluid and is often patted dry with a soft cloth right at birth for warmth. Its skin is soft to the touch and usually very smooth. It may be somewhat wrinkly from its life in the amniotic fluid if it is born early or late.

- *Skin color:* Your baby's skin will be pink all over, or possibly blue on the hands and feet at first. Pink color shows strong blood circulation; bluish color, that circulation is building up. The skin of babies of nonwhite parents usually has not achieved its full pigmentation at birth.

- *Creamy vernix on the skin:* Your baby will probably arrive with at least some natural cream on his or her skin. Called vernix, it serves as a protective substance through pregnancy and may be largely worn off by the amniotic fluid before birth. The baby's skin gradually absorbs the vernix after birth, so it may be advisable to wash it off gently only where it is especially thick—as in the creases of the skin in the groin and armpits, or possibly mixed in with the baby's hair on the scalp.

- *No hair, or thick hair:* It's perfectly normal for babies to be born with little or no hair or, on the other hand, with a thick head of hair. Also, the color of the hair often changes after it grows for a few weeks or months—perhaps from black to brown or even blond. Some babies are born with fine, downy soft, dark hair on parts of their bodies (face, shoulders, back, upper arms, and legs). Called lanugo, it is more likely to be seen on premature babies and falls out over the first week or so after birth.

- *Dark spots on the back:* Some babies of black or Latin parents are born with one or more small black areas on their lower backs or buttocks. These fade away in time. They are not bruises or blemishes.

- *Molding and soft spots on the head:* As you can see in the birth illustrations in the preceding chapter the still-soft bones of the baby's head are shaped as they pass through the birth canal. This molding usually gives an elongated look to a newborn's head, and may cause the head to bulge a bit in one direction or another. Such elongation and bulging after a typical normal birth represent no harm whatever to the infant. Within a day or two it will correct itself and the baby's head will look normally rounded.

Two openings between the baby's skull bones, called fontanelles, allowed the baby's head to mold during birth. These are spaces where the bones have not yet grown together. They're on the center line of the head, straight up from the nose. The frontal one (anterior fontanelle) is located on top of the head, above the forehead, and the rear one (posterior fontanelle) is much smaller and is found at the occiput (the highest part of your head when you rest your chin on your chest).

Incidentally, identifying the location of these fontanelles by vaginal examination during labor enables a maternity care-giver to determine the position of the fetus in the uterus.

These soft spots on the head will be filled in by bone growth before the baby's second birthday. Usually the posterior one fills in by the age of 6 weeks to 2 months; the anterior one, by 15 to 18 months. Until they do fill in, you should be especially careful to keep anything from pressing on the baby's head at those points even though a tough membrane covers the opening between bones.

• *Head and neck movements:* At birth your baby can turn its head from side to side. And if placed lying down on its tummy, the baby's neck muscles have the strength to lift its head up.

However, when you hold the baby on its back, you need to be sure to support the back of its head. The baby's neck muscles do not yet have the strength to keep its head from sagging backward or rolling from side to side.

One popular way of carrying the baby is to hold it snugly against your chest with one hand supporting the back of its head and the other hand holding its buttocks. Another way is to carry the baby with a one-handed "football carry," much as players carry the ball for security against fumbling. In this, the baby lies on its back on your forearm, held level with its head resting on the upturned hand of that arm. You keep it tucked snugly against your side, your upper arm in a straight line down from your shoulder. The opposite hand is then free.

• *Disproportionately large genital organs:* Newborns have genital organs that are large in proportion to their size. For a day or two female and boy newborns may secrete small amounts of milk from slightly enlarged breasts as a result of the same hormonal stimulation that causes engorgement and milk production in their mothers.

Female babies may in some cases have a white mucuslike vaginal discharge that may be tinged with blood. This also results from the mother's hormones. It passes in a day or so. Use baby oil and be gentle in cleaning the discharge.

Apgar Scoring

Currently, the accepted form of evaluating your baby's overall condition is through an Apgar score at one and five minutes after the birth. Five areas of observation, heart rate, respiration, muscle tone, reflexes and skin color, are scored on a scale of 0 to 2 each, so that the highest possible total score is 10. A score of 7 or more generally indicates satisfactory condition. Scores lower than 7 indicate that one or more of the baby's systems need help in order to work properly—most commonly the respiratory system.

Other measures to ensure your baby's health are taken, but do not need to be performed in the first minute after birth. These include:

Silver Nitrate or Antibiotic Ointment in the Eyes: Health department regulations in many states require that babies be given 1 percent silver nitrate solution drops in the eyes shortly after birth. (Antibiotic ointment may be used instead in some states, including California, New York, and Oregon.) This prevents blindness should there be a gonorrheal infection in the birth canal at the time of an infant's birth. Erythromycin offers broader spectrum prophylaxis (against chlamydia, for example) than does silver nitrate, and it has been recommended by the American Academy of Pediatrics.

Eye drops or ointment do blur the infant's vision temporarily. Parents and care-givers accordingly delay eye treatment for an hour or so after birth so that the infant can have full vision during the bonding process.

You should discuss any preferences or questions concerning this requirement with your birth-care or pediatric-care provider.

Vitamin K Injection: A single vitamin K injection is also often given to the newborn by your care-provider as a precautionary measure. The purpose is to facilitate bloodclotting, since newborns cannot synthesize vitamin K until they develop the necessary intestinal bacteria to do so, which occurs a few days after birth.

Parents can request that the vitamin K injection be omitted. Some parents think the injection is needlessly upsetting to the baby and believe that enough vitamin K is provided through the mother's system if she is breastfeeding. In addition, they think that the vitamin K may add to the possibility that an infant may develop jaundice. If you do not want this injection to be given, discuss the benefits and risks with your pediatric care-provider.

Other Quick Checkups and Records: Care-givers take your fingerprints and the baby's footprints for required essential identification. They also record your baby's temperature (with a rectal thermometer, checking also to be sure the rectum has no obstructions), weight in pounds and ounces (and in grams), head-to-heel length in inches, and the diameter of the largest part of the baby's head and chest.

The condition or functioning of other parts of the baby's body will also be checked, including ears, chest, breasts, shoulder blades, shoulder and jaw and hip joints, heart, lungs, and the abdomen (including the liver, spleen, and kidneys).

A blood sample will be taken from the umbilical cord for blood tests. Care-givers will also watch to make sure that soon after birth your baby urinates and has a first bowel movement (which consists of a sticky, tarry substance called meconium).

Your Health Care Right after Birth

After the birth, your care-givers will assist as needed to make sure the placenta is expelled in third-stage labor. Your pelvic floor will be examined, and it will be sutured if it has sustained a tear while being stretched by the baby's birth, or if you have been given an episiotomy. A local anesthetic like Novocain will be given for the suturing.

Your uterus will be checked for firmness. You can also do this yourself by putting your hand on your abdomen at the level of your navel and pressing down in various locations to see if your uterus feels firm. Your abdomen, now flat, will be soft and flabby after having been stretched for so long. (Exercises can firm and tone it.)

Your uterus will be about the size of a grapefruit. As you massage it, it will become very firm, even hard, and you may notice a gush of fluid from your vagina. This postnatal vaginal discharge, called lochia, will be watched to see that it doesn't reach levels that might indicate hemorrhaging (heavy internal bleeding). At the start, the lochia will be bright red and intermittent.

Care-givers may apply ice packs to your pelvic floor tissues if they're swollen from the strain of birth.

Your blood pressure, pulse, and temperature will be taken. You and your support partner will be urged to eat and drink for nourishment after your hard work. Once you've started to breastfeed, and after you've all started to bond and have rested a bit, your partner can help you take a shower if you're at a birth center or at home. Next, you might all celebrate with a festive meal and then get more rest.

First Several Hours after Birth

After those busy first hours of your baby's life, your pediatrician will make a first examination if you're at a birth center or hospital. (The center's or hospital's own pediatrician may do this initial examination.) You may find this a welcome time to talk over with the pediatrician any questions you have about the baby or about caring for it.

You and your partner should feel free to hold and cuddle your newborn as much as you like in these first few hours. Children who have been at or near the birth can join in this bonding. Holding and cuddling the new baby can give your children an important feeling of closeness and affection.

Let the baby nurse as much as you both like. Desirable bonding and nursing like this can be done naturally by having your baby stay with you all the time at a birth center, or by "rooming-in" at a hospital.

If you are at a hospital, tell care-givers that you want your baby to nurse like this (called demand feeding) rather than letting them give the baby water from a bottle in between nursings. Such bottle feedings are frequently given in hospitals, because of a concern about minor dehydration and low blood sugar levels in newborns. These feedings are not needed by the healthy babies of well-nourished mothers, and they do interfere with getting breastfeeding off to a good start.

Sugar water or plain water bottle feedings for your baby are all right if you do not plan to breastfeed. It would still be a good idea to breastfeed colostrum to your newborn for two or three feedings right after birth. Doing so will provide immunities for the baby, help shrink your uterus, promote bonding, and comfort the infant, as discussed before.

You should enjoy giving your baby its bottle feedings with as much loving care as if you were breastfeeding. A formula will be recommended for continued bottlefeeding after you go home, and you will receive instructions for preparing it.

Rest for you, your baby, and your partner will be a top priority in these first few hours. You may find yourself keenly excited, alert, and energetic for many hours after the birth. A number of new mothers feel this way, possibly as a result of hormonal action. It's still advisable to sit or lie down much of the time and to take nourishment in order to restore your energy and strength. It is also sensible to limit visitors to your home until your strength returns and your new routines are established.

You and your baby will find yourselves ready to take up family life at home in a surprisingly short time if you've had a normal birth

244

experience. In view of this, birth centers allow you to go home within twelve hours postpartum. Some birth-center families take their new babies home even earlier.

Hospitals today are also encouraging increasingly early discharge after normal birth. Discharge after two or three days has become fairly common, and some hospitals are allowing mothers to return home within twenty-four hours of birth.

Circumcision

In the past, circumcision was very commonly done before the mother and baby left the hospital. Whether or not to have your baby circumcised has recently become a more controversial question. Some 90 percent or more of all male babies in this country were circumcised during the 1950s and 1960s. Rising opposition to the practice resulted in a decrease to 75 percent by 1980.

Parents whose religion historically requires circumcision understandably find that this reason outweighs all others. For other parents, circumcision is done mainly for these reasons: the belief that in later life it contributes to lower incidence of cancer of the penis or the cervix of the man's mate; the belief that circumcision improves personal hygiene; and the desire to have the boy's penis look like the majority of other boys' penises (or to look like his dad's), and to go along with a practice accepted unquestioningly by many parents and groups.

Parents who oppose having their babies circumcised are against it mainly for these reasons:

- It does not seem to be related to lower incidence of cancer of the penis or of the cervix. This idea was based on the fact that there is a low incidence of such cancer among Jewish families, but later analyses showed that the low incidence was attributable to lower rates of sexual promiscuity among Jewish families.

- It causes needless pain for the newborn (circumcision is usually done without anesthesia of any kind because anesthetics are harmful to infants).

- Circumcision is not essential for personal hygiene in this day and time.

- Increasing numbers of boys are not being circumcised; therefore, uncircumcised boys will not feel different, particularly as the practice continues to decrease in years ahead.

If You're Having a Traditional Hospital Birth

A family-centered hospital birth experience is likely to be much the same as described in this chapter.

If you're having a traditional hospital birth, differences will include not having the baby with you as much, and not having your support partner present with you and the baby most of the time.

After a traditional hospital birth, your partner will remain in a visitors' waiting room. Your baby will be shown to you briefly in the delivery room. It will then be taken to the hospital nursery, where all newborns are cared for except for brief feeding periods with their mothers.

Your partner can visit you after you return to your hospital room. He will see the baby only through the nursery window. He will not usually be allowed to stay with you when the baby is brought to your room for feeding. This is done mainly in order to avoid risk of infection. Such risk has been found to be slight or nonexistent in other settings, however.

You and your baby will usually stay in the hospital for three or four days before going home. Such hospital stays may be related to the recovery from drugs used in labor and at birth. During the hospital stay, classes on infant care and feeding may be provided. Take advantage of them if they are offered by your hospital.

15

The Baby's First Few Weeks

Babies need to be hugged and held a great deal. Their skin and sense of touch are far more sensitive than those of an adult. This acute sensitivity can result in blotches and outbreaks of tiny rashes from the least irritation, but it also helps the baby learn about its environment.

As a result, your baby is not merely soothed by gentleness, warmth, stroking, cuddling, and steady rocking while being held and hugged—it is being stimulated in its development. Numbers of studies have shown that babies whose needs for physical contact and touching are regularly satisfied show more rapid neurological and mental development and greater weight gain than other babies. So, hold the baby as much as possible; don't worry about "spoiling" a newborn.

In addition, you need the experience of cuddling and hugging the baby almost as much for your own emotional satisfaction. The more cuddling and hugging you do, the more at home you'll feel with the baby.

Physical contact between the baby and its father is also very important. At the Childbearing Center the fathers too go through the bonding process with their newborns. They report that they enjoy holding, caring for, and playing wholeheartedly with their babies. Doing so helps them feel comfortable and rounds out their own personal development. Moreover, fathers can serve as uniquely valuable sources of affection for their infants. Babies thrive on attention and warmth from their fathers, as well as from all other family members.

Getting Your Baby Settled

With the new baby in your home, you'll start shifting to new patterns of daily life. Key aspects of those patterns concern what the baby needs most—feeding and related care like diaper-changing, getting enough sleep, and the relief of other needs often expressed by crying.

Feeding

Continue the pattern you've established for feeding your baby. You'll already have learned much about breastfeeding or bottlefeeding from your prenatal or hospital postpartum classes, and possibly from meetings of a local La Leche League group, as discussed in Chapter 11.

Diaper-Changing, Urination, and Bowel Movements

Your baby will be wearing disposable or cloth diapers starting almost from birth. Check to see that he or she starts urinating within the first twenty-four hours. Even though the baby is not taking in much fluid, newborns excrete fluid they retained in their tissues during uterine life. Six to eight wet diapers a day indicate that your baby is well hydrated.

Once feeding is better established after the first few days, you can expect even more wet diapers a day. Again, this indicates that the baby is getting enough fluids.

A baby's urine is clear or pale yellow. During the first week it may leave a reddish stain resembling brick dust on the diaper. This is temporary and normal, but if it persists, check with your baby's care-provider.

A black tarry substance called meconium comprises the first bowel movements of the newborn. Your baby should have a bowel movement within twenty-four hours of birth. You can wash off the meconium most easily with warm water or baby oil.

If you have a girl, when cleansing her after a bowel movement, always wipe from front to back to avoid spreading any possible bacteria from the anal area to the vaginal or urethral areas.

The stools of a breastfed baby usually change in the first few days from greenish brown to yellow-green or yellow, and have a liquid or pasty consistency. At times they may contain curdlike lumps mixed with liquid material. On occasion the stool may be a little more than a stain on the diaper. It has no unpleasant odor, and the baby is seldom if ever constipated. Bowel movements may come after every feeding, or only once every few days; either pattern is normal.

For a bottlefed baby, the stools change from meconium to yellow or yellow-brown in color. They are soft to pasty in consistency, but much more formed and solid than those of a breastfed baby. Your bottlefed baby may have two to four bowel movements daily. Dry or hard stools usually indicate a need for more water. Offer a nursing bottle of water to the baby a couple of times a day to make sure he or she gets enough liquid. Sometimes an adjustment in the formula may be needed as well. Always check with your baby's care-provider before making any changes.

Hiccups and Spitting Up

Even though you've helped your baby to bring up burps of swallowed air during a feeding, the baby may get spells of hiccups from time to time. They sound loud and shake the baby's whole body. But vigorous hiccups like these are normal and do not seem to bother most babies. Hiccups usually stop spontaneously in a short time. By the time the baby is 3 months old, these spells of hiccups occur much less often.

Frequently little spit-ups of milk are also perfectly normal. They occur even after you've faithfully burped the baby. They may be caused by a little mucus in the mouth or throat. They may also be caused by overfeeding. But the main explanation is that the sphincter muscles of the baby's stomach are still immature and milk regurgitates easily. Most often, as the baby gets older these muscles strengthen and spitting up decreases.

However, frequently forceful spitting up of larger amounts of milk after feedings may indicate a health problem. Tell your baby's caregiver if you think the amount of milk seems large and is more like vomiting than spitting up.

Sleeping Patterns

Babies just a few days old have natural sleeping patterns that vary widely. Consider yourself very lucky if your baby is one of the few who sleeps after nighttime feedings and is awake and playful between naps during daytime hours. Usually newborn babies wake every two or three hours (or more often) for feedings around the clock, but they will often have one four- or five-hour-long sleep at some time during each twenty-four hours.

Babies can thrive even though they may sleep only twelve hours or less out of every twenty-four hours. Babies can also thrive if they sleep mostly during the days while staying awake through the night. If your baby tends to stay awake at night, these suggestions will help protect your health while guiding your baby toward nighttime sleeping.

- If you can, you should sleep when the baby sleeps, in order to protect your strength. Try to get household help for routine chores as needed to do this.

- Every two or three hours during the day, offer the baby a feeding even if you need to wake the baby gently in order to do so. Drowsy babies will often wake up enough for a feeding if they're somewhat hungry. If the baby will not feed, do not force the issue.

- Through the evenings, play with the baby and continue to try to feed it every two or three hours. Doing so should help tire the baby for sleeping at night.

- Also give the baby a bath in the evening rather than in the morning.

- Keep nighttime feeding periods just for feedings and diaper-changings. Playing with the baby may stimulate wakefulness. After feeding, changing, and burping, put the baby into his or her bed to encourage going back to sleep. (Understand, though, that this type of "scheduling" is not realistic in the first month or so. It may work better when the baby is about 2 or 3 months old. Even then, it may not. Some babies are 4 to 6 months old, or older, before they sleep through the night on a fairly regular basis.)

Crying

In normal babies hunger most often causes crying. As a result, you should assume that your baby is hungry whenever it cries, unless another need is very obviously the case, and be ready to feed the baby without delay at any hour of the day or night. (Such readiness represents one of the main advantages of breastfeeding.)

When your baby wakes up crying and could possibly be hungry, start feeding it right away without stopping to change its diaper or otherwise delay the feeding. Hunger is apparently sharply painful to babies. They are usually impatient to be fed. Holding off too long on the feeding while doing something else may make the baby too overwrought or too worn out to feed properly. You can diaper or dress the baby during breaks in the feeding to burp or change positions.

Your baby's crying tells you of any discomfort or distress—including hunger—that he or she is feeling. In some cases the crying spell is short and stops by itself. This can happen just before the baby urinates, passes some gas, or has a bowel movement, for instance. But in most cases you should try to relieve the cause of the crying by comforting or otherwise helping the baby. In addition to having some physical distress, your baby may cry because it feels frightened, lonely, deserted, tired, or just bored.

Fussing: Babies usually have a regular time every day when they fuss by crying lightly off and on and otherwise acting restless. Unfortunately, this fussy time often comes in the evenings.

Hold and talk to the baby if you can during these fussy periods. Being cuddled, stroked, and talked to softly comforts most babies. You can help your baby through these fussy periods by responding with love to cries for attention and care. Doing so also strengthens the baby's trust in its world and helps build its future sense of self-confidence.

An after-dinner fussy time might be dealt with by a ride in the baby carriage or the family car. Or after it can control its head your baby might enjoy being rocked or sung to while held up high on your shoulder, or on its father's shoulder, so it can see all around. Some babies also like to lie tummy down across a lap.

Should fussy periods arrive while you have to get dinner or look after an older child, you might use a baby carrier in order to hold the baby close to your chest and leave your hands free (the type of carriers made of heavy denim or other strong, canvas-like cloth). The baby can be held fully supported against your chest and can feel the reassuring beat of your heart and the vibration of your voice.

Fear-caused crying: Babies may also cry when startled by a sudden loud noise. Sounds like a door slamming, a doorbell ringing, or a dog barking can alarm your baby and trigger crying (with perhaps the sudden body-jerk of the baby's startle reflex coming first). If such alarms do make your baby cry, hold the baby close to you and talk to her or him softly and reassuringly until the panic is over.

Pain-caused crying: On rare occasions, babies will cry because of pain—typically the pain of gas or an ache in the stomach. When feeling such pain the baby will often arch its back, pull up its legs, and refuse to be fed or soothed. These are the symptoms of colic, a condition of apparent digestive disturbance which usually goes away at 3 months of age. Although colic occurs with less frequency in breastfed babies, any infant may be a colicky baby.

In a case like this, first see if you can burp the baby and thus relieve stomach gas. If that doesn't work, try to rock or walk with the baby in different positions. The pain of a stomach cramp will often ease away after you simply hold and comfort the baby for a while. Sometimes the baby is constipated, which can be relieved by gently inserting a rectal thermometer coated with petroleum jelly to stimulate the passage of fecal material and gas. The tummy down position on a warm heating pad may help. But often nothing seems to relieve colic and attacks recur over the first three months.

Fatigue-caused crying: You may also run into times when the baby goes on crying for no apparent reason—no hunger, no need for a diaper change, no itch from a diaper rash, no stomachache, no constipation, no loneliness, and no fever or other sign indicating illness. This may mean simply that the baby is tired, or maybe even overtired.

Go on rocking or holding the baby for a while longer and see if it doesn't drop off to sleep. Or you might try putting the baby into its crib, making it thoroughly comfortable with covers, favorite toys, and a loving pat, and letting it try to go off to sleep. It may cry loudly for a short time, then stop crying, cry a little more off and on, and finally sink into slumber.

If the baby is still crying: Here are some other practical measures that experienced mothers use to comfort babies who are still crying after being fed and changed, rocked and hugged, checked and inspected:

• Try swaddling. Some babies feel more secure when snugly wrapped. Also, it diminishes the startle reflex.

• Try a pacifier (preferably one that is orthodontically designed). Giving a pacifier on occasion doesn't make you a negligent parent. At times babies may want to suck but not be hungry. Some babies have a very strong sucking drive, and giving them a pacifier helps to satisfy it.

• Try motion, taking a ride in the stroller, carriage, or a car. This may help particularly at bedtime. If they're at all tired, some babies find sleep irresistible in a car.

• Try turning on the radio or TV. This might soothe your baby if she or he is one who doesn't like the house to be too quiet.

• Try running the vacuum cleaner. That steady noise really does quiet some crying babies.

• You might try music, or perhaps a commercially available phonograph record that features the sounds of a mother's body and heartbeat. Or you could just put the baby on your tummy and chest instead, in case the baby prefers hearing the real thing.

Responding now means less crying later: During the first weeks of your baby's life—indeed, through the first year—try to meet the baby's needs as soon as possible to avoid excessive crying. At this age it's impossible to spoil the baby with too much love and attention.

A number of studies have shown that babies whose needs have been promptly met in the early months of life are less and less demanding as they grow older. Other studies have shown that frequent crying by normal babies ends after a surprisingly short time. Babies start crying for substantial amounts of time when they're about 3 weeks old, when they build up to a total of two to four hours a day. After that, crying time diminishes and has very largely ended by the age of only 12 weeks.

Getting Yourselves Started as New Parents

Get Enough Rest

During your baby's first few weeks, remember that you can't take good care of the baby unless you first take care of yourself. And at the start your most critical need is rest.

Make your main activities simply caring for the baby and yourself. If you're breastfeeding, rest much or most of the time until after your milk comes in and your baby is well established in nursing. (Your milk should come in about the second or third day after birth, if you're feeding on demand and nursing will be established in three to four weeks.

Make your only other activities moments of close affection with your partner, and some short times of undivided attention for your other children.

Otherwise, prohibit visitors (unless they come to help in specific ways that you designate), neglect housework, and ignore hobbies for the time being.

Get Homemaking Help if Feasible

Have someone help you at home through the first week or two, if you possibly can. Your helper should be a person you're completely comfortable with—for example, the baby's father if time permits, your mother or mother-in-law if the relationship is congenial, any relative or friend you like, or a paid homemaker if funds permit. In the case of a hired homemaker, be sure to meet the person before the baby's birth to avoid unpleasant surprises later. Try not to pick someone whose ways are so different from your own that it will be a strain just to have the person around.

A helper might relieve you by preparing meals, doing food shopping, caring for an older child, doing housecleaning and laundry, and diapering, bathing, holding, and playing with the baby.

It's no cause for panic if you can't arrange for a helper. Take on only what you can comfortably handle beyond feeding and caring for the baby, and let anything else go.

Energy-Saving Measures

Watch for ways to conserve your energy. For example, designate an area for baby care that's conveniently located, perhaps by your bed. Organize the baby articles so that you don't have to stoop, reach, or leave the baby to find them. A rolling utility cart or serving table with wheels to move food, dishes, supplies, or clothes from one room to another can save trips back and forth.

Guard against overexerting yourself in the baby's first few weeks. Avoid climbing stairs if you can. If you can't, take them slowly enough to avoid feeling pushed.

Do not lift heavy objects by bending over, at least for the first few weeks. Keep your back straight and crouch down by bending your knees if you absolutely must lift. With a toddler, sit on a couch or chair and let the child climb up onto your lap instead of lifting him or her from the floor. (p. 93)

Teamwork as a Couple

Having worked together through the prenatal preparations and the birth itself, you and your partner should find it not only natural but rewarding to work together in caring for your new baby. The first few weeks or months may bring times when you both feel exhausted or worried about the baby. Help and understanding from each other can make an enormous difference. Being able to give or get such help when needed becomes easier if you and your partner keep communications open and try to meet each other's needs.

Your Older Children

The needs of your other children deserve your attention as well. Remember to let your child know that you and your partner care about him or her just as much as ever. The warmth and sincerity with which you do this counts much more than the time it may take to do so.

Building a sense of your family caring for one another reinforces the good feelings older children have about themselves and the new baby. Watching you and your partner give each other emotional support while caring for the baby can strengthen the sense of love and security they have about their family.

Getting children accustomed to daily routines with a baby in the home may not be easy. But older children, if treated gently and considerately, will in time feel good about having a baby sister or brother in their lives. If they were able to be present at the birth (or had minimal separation from you at that time), the adjustment will very likely be easier. And remember to include them in care just as you did in the preparations.

Caring for Your Own Needs

Personal Hygiene

You may get sweats at night or at other times as your body gradually gets rid of excess fluid accumulation in the first few days after birth. Take showers as needed—they can feel especially refreshing. Tub baths are all right if you had no stitches or perineal/vaginal tears. Wait to take a tub bath until three or four days after the birth if you have an episiotomy or stitches.

With stitches from either a tear or an episiotomy, cleanse the area after you urinate or have a bowel movement by pouring warm tap water from a plastic squeeze bottle over the area and blotting it dry with soft tissue.

After the third or fourth day you can sit in a bath of warm water only about 2 or 3 inches deep, for about ten to fifteen minutes. These sitz baths may be continued until healing is complete.

Soreness of the sutured area can be relieved and healing promoted by exposing it to the heat of a 40-watt bulb placed about 12 to 18 inches from the area for ten to fifteen minutes three times a day.

Vaginal Discharge

Expect a fairly heavy vaginal discharge, called lochia, in the days following birth. At first it will be heavier than your normal menstrual flow, and bright red. Gradually it will change to a pinkish and then a yellowish color, and finally become white. The flow may occur for some three to five weeks and will be intermittent rather than steady. Use feminine napkins rather than tampons.

You may feel an increased flow when the baby nurses if you're breastfeeding, because nursing causes the uterus to contract, expelling any collected blood and tissue debris. Your flow may also increase when you rise from a sitting or lying position (due simply to the emptying out of lochia pooled in the vagina).

Too much exertion can cause the flow to increase and the bright red color to return or persist. If you see this, or if you pass blood clots, you should call your care-giver, ask advice, and decrease your activities.

When your baby is about 3 weeks old, you may have what seems like a light menstrual period for a day or two. This is actually the final part of the uterine lining to which the placenta had been attached. The resulting bright red flow will slow down after a day or two, and the discharge will go back to what it had been like before this episode.

Urination and Bowel Movements

Don't be surprised if you continue to urinate as often after birth as before labor started. This may occur while your bladder is getting back in condition and your body is excreting excess fluid accumulated in late pregnancy.

To promote easy, regular bowel movements, drink juices and other fluids frequently in the early days after birth, and eat abundant roughage such as salads, bran, fruits, and vegetables.

Relax when trying to move your bowels. Do not worry that it will cause your stitches to break. Avoid using laxatives unless really essential. Ask for advice from your health-care-giver if you haven't had a bowel movement by the third day after birth.

Care of the Breasts

If you're breastfeeding: Special fullness, hardness, and tenderness of the breasts usually develops after the milk comes in on the second to fourth day. This is called engorgement. Its severity varies from woman to woman, and it lasts only two to four days.

Nursing the baby frequently relieves engorgement without further remedies. But if you still need relief, or if the fullness makes it hard for your baby to grasp the nipple, try softening the breasts before nursing by wrapping them in a warm, wet towel for several minutes or by taking a warm shower.

Also, you can soften the areola (the dark area around the nipple) by expressing a small amount of milk before the baby nurses.

Other suggestions include:

Do not wash your nipples before nursing. They're kept clean by oily secretions from glands on the areola (called Montgomery tubercles).

When taking a bath or shower, use only plain water to wash your breasts; soap can dry and irritate the nipples.

Change the nursing pads whenever they are wet, as well as the bra itself if it also becomes wet. (This also decreases the chance of developing sore nipples.)

At the start of breastfeeding, nipples tend to feel tender and sore until the baby's nursing makes them less sensitive after a few days. If your nipples feel uncomfortably sore after feedings, you can speed the desensitizing process in these ways:

- Leave the nipples exposed to the air for fifteen to twenty minutes after each feeding by leaving nursing bra flaps down or by removing your bra.

- Expose the nipples to sunlight (be careful about direct exposure) for three to five minutes at a time; or instead, expose them for three to five minutes to the heat given off by a 40-watt incandescent light bulb placed 12 to 18 inches away from the breasts.

- Apply lanolin, a mild ointment, vitamin E oil, or some of your own milk to the nipples after you wash and dry the breasts. Use very little cream or oil so that none remains on the surface after you gently work the substance into the nipple and areola. There is no need to wash before the baby's next feeding.

To keep soreness to a minimum, give the baby short, frequent feedings that provide adequate milk flow and satisfy the baby's hunger in the shortest sucking time. Let the baby nurse first on the nipple that feels less sore, because your initial "let-down" reflex will ease the milk flow from the more sore breast, and your baby will not have to suck as vigorously to get the milk.

Keep a glass of water or juice handy in case you feel very thirsty just as the let-down comes and your milk starts to flow.

If you're bottlefeeding: Until your breasts go back to their original size, wear a support bra while you sleep as well as through the day. Marked swelling (engorgement) of the breasts will occur on the second to the fourth day. It should subside in another day or two.

During engorgement, continue to wear a support bra (or bind your breasts so that they are supported) to promote good circulation, provide comfort, and reduce swelling. To relieve discomfort from engorgement, you can apply ice packs to the breasts over your bra. Taking aspirin (or an aspirin substitute) may also help. Do not try to express milk to ease the discomfort; it will only increase the milk supply.

You probably won't need to take medicine containing hormones to relieve engorgement. These medications are best avoided if possible.

A whitish yellow or orange-yellow fluid may continue to leak from your nipples from time to time for a few weeks. It will cease gradually as your milk dries up completely and your breasts regain their prepregnancy size.

Mood Swings

Your hormones are readjusting to new levels in the days following birth. These shifts may cause your moods to swing up or down, from elation to depression. As a result, you may find yourself crying at times for no reason at all, or you may laugh more than usual when something funny occurs. If you happen to get highly erratic reactions like these, tell others around you—and yourself—that you're sorry, but it's just your hormones getting back in balance. Hormonal adjustments and adjustment to parenthood sometimes combine to make these mood swings rather intense at times. Realize that for most women this is a temporary, albeit difficult, time—but it will pass.

Resuming Intercourse

Wait to have intercourse again until you've stopped bleeding and feel comfortable about it—psychologically as well as physically. Judging by these criteria seems to work better than adhering to the arbitrary six weeks after the birth that was advised by many physicians in past years.

Two suggestions for the first few times you resume intercourse: (1) Go easy on the physical intensity, for you may feel somewhat sore and tender. (2) Have a water-based vaginal lubricating jelly or contraceptive cream on hand, in case you want to use it. (Do not use petroleum jelly.) Some women experience less natural lubrication than usual in the first few weeks after birth and the early months of breastfeeding. The lubricating secretions almost always increase with time.

Even after the birth of a large baby, the vagina resumes a smaller size than before pregnancy for a number of women. Such tightness often eases once ovulation starts again.

You can ovulate and hence become pregnant as early as four to six weeks after birth. Although this is not usual, it is possible. If you want to avoid pregnancy, you should use some form of contraception when you resume intercourse. Using both condoms and contraceptive foam can give you reasonably adequate protection at the outset. You could later use whichever form of contraception you prefer—diaphragm or contraceptive pill among them—after having a medical checkup and discussing choices with your care-provider.

Breastfeeding will affect your options, eliminating the pill for a few months. Some care-providers do not favor the IUD for any woman. Also, your partner could continue to use condoms though it's best if you also use foam; contraception should not be solely the woman's responsibility.

Checkups after the Birth

If you had your baby at a birth center, you will usually be examined at home during the first week (by their staff or a public health nurse) and at the center one week after the birth. The professional caregiver who attended you at the birth will do the one-week examination if possible. A similar postnatal (or postpartum) examination for followup purposes would typically be done five to six weeks after birth.

If you had your baby at a hospital, the six-week postpartum examination would probably be the only one offered as a regular part of childbirth services.

You will have to arrange for any additional health care or treatment you need. Such care could be given either by the same professional, or by other physicians or care-givers you select.

Exercises

Two types of exercises are very important after birth. To help tone and flatten your abdomen, do the head and shoulders lift exercise described in Chapter 10. Start with five lifts each morning and night, and increase by one lift per day until you are doing twenty each morning and night.

Kegel exercises, for toning the muscles of your pelvic floor, are the second type of especially important exercises after birth. Resume these as soon as you feel somewhat rested, preferably within twenty-four hours of birth. Kegels are valuable exercises for all adult women to do throughout life for good pelvic floor condition, as explained in Chapter 10. In resuming them, gradually build up to the level of at least fifty a day, as you did during pregnancy.

Health clubs, dance studios, yoga centers, and "Y" programs sponsor special exercise classes for women who have recently given birth. These could be extremely effective in conditioning your body. Make sure you're in sufficiently good health before you start, though. In general, hold off until you have had your five-to-six-week check and verify also with your care-provider.

Some classes offer a baby-sitting service. If you use one of these, try to schedule your classes for times when the baby is least likely to be hungry or fussy.

Your Baby's Care

Washing and Bathing

Use a soft cloth or cotton ball to wash these parts of the baby every day:

- face and neck (and folds in the neck),
- behind the ears (especially to get any spit-up milk that may have collected there), and
- genitalia and buttocks (which you should wash both daily and after each bowel movement).

If a diaper rash starts to develop, apply a light coating of baby ointment or petroleum jelly to the reddish patches and nearby areas. It will help soothe and protect the sensitive skin. Expose the diaper area to air as much as possible. Place waterproof pads under the baby when you do.

Your baby can get along perfectly well without having a full bath until it is a week or more old. Besides, you should wait for the navel to heal completely (and the circumcised penis, if circumcision was done). You can then give the baby a bath daily or every few days as you prefer.

Shampoo your baby's hair at the same time you give regular baths, and gently but thoroughly massage the scalp while shampooing.

After rinsing, gently but vigorously rub the baby's scalp with a soft bath towel. Drying it like this and following up with a good brushing and combing (if the baby has very long hair) stimulates the scalp. It also helps prevent "cradle cap," scaly patches that are oily and grayish yellow and are often hard to remove once they accumulate. A little baby oil or special commercial product (as suggested by your pediatric care-giver) helps loosen these patches, so they can be combed or brushed out more easily.

Umbilical Cord Care

No special washing is needed for the umbilical cord stump before it dries up and falls off by itself, any time from about four days to two weeks after birth. Dry it gently after washing around it. Keep it exposed to the air by folding the diaper below it and the shirt above it.

When the stump comes off, you may see a drop of blood on the navel. If so, or if the navel looks a little moist then or later, apply rubbing alcohol once or twice a day with a cotton ball (to help promote healing) and leave it open to the air.

Eye Care

For the first few days there might be a small amount of mucuslike discharge on the baby's eyelids. This is a common reaction to the silver nitrate drops that are often put in babies' eyes at birth. If it does occur, wipe the discharge away gently from each eye with a separate moistened cotton ball to prevent a crust from forming.

In some instances a newborn baby will have a small red spot or two on the eyeball, the result of the rupture of a tiny blood vessel during birth. They disappear in time.

Jaundice

Jaundice arises in babies from a buildup of bilirubin (yellow bile pigments) in the skin, which is caused by the breakdown of excess red blood cells that were needed before birth. The baby's liver has not yet matured enough to dispose of the bilirubin quickly. Blood tests may be needed to measure the exact bilirubin level if your baby has more than a mild case.

Mild, nonharmful jaundice occurs in more than half of all babies born after normal full-term pregnancies. These cases usually begin on about the second or third day after birth and clear up spontaneously after five to nine days.

If you think your baby might have jaundice, look for these signs:

- Yellow color in the whites of the baby's eyes.
- Yellowish color in the baby's skin (look at the baby in the daylight, by a window. The skin may look slightly tanned or have a peachlike color.) Gently press on the baby's nose or breastbone: jaundiced skin looks yellowish rather than blanching when you release the pressure.

- Yellowish color in the palms of the baby's hands and the soles of its feet.
- Accompanying fever, drowsiness, or lack of appetite.

Notify your pediatric care-giver right away if you see one or more of these signs. If not monitored carefully, jaundice can become severe and possibly harmful.

Your care-giver may instruct you to try to prevent or help clear up mild jaundice in several ways. In warm sunny weather, take the baby's clothes off (except perhaps for the diaper), and expose its skin to sunlight for *no more than* two to five minutes at a time. Or you may be told to have the baby sleep in indirect sunlight near a window with as much skin exposed as possible. The blue light rays in sunlight cause a breakdown of the bilirubin in the skin through photo-oxidation into safe by-products. Be sure to follow your care-giver's instructions faithfully if you use natural sunlight for phototherapy.

If you are breastfeeding, try to nurse the baby often (as much as every couple of hours). Frequent nursing is effective because colostrum and breast milk stimulate the baby's intestines to eliminate bilirubin. You can also give the baby a bottle of water several times a day.

If your baby needs further treatment, your physician will put it under a special lamp in the hospital, which simulates sunlight but can be controlled more effectively. Your baby might need this photo-therapy for one or two days. Ask about lamps for use at home.

When to Phone Your Pediatric Care-Giver

Trust yourself to care for your baby's basic needs. However, some conditions warrant checking with your pediatrician, family physician, or nurse-practitioner to see if professional help is needed. Phone your baby's professional care-giver for advice about any of these conditions:

- No passage of urine or meconium within twenty-four hours after birth.
- Fewer than four or five wet diapers in any twenty-four-hour period after the baby's second day.
- A yellowish or sun-tanned color indicating jaundice. Report even what appears to be mild jaundice, though it may need no corrective measures.
- Vomiting of what looks like an entire feeding, especially if forcefully expelled.
- Signs of infection around the navel such as swelling, redness, a rash, oozing, or a foul smell.

- Fever, as indicated by a temperature (taken with a rectal thermometer) higher than the normal rectal temperature of 99.6°. *Definitely* report fever of 100.6° or over.

- Any other signs that strongly suggest your baby is not well (even if there is no fever), including a different sound to the baby's crying; listlessness, or lack of usual movement and liveliness by the baby; vomiting; a marked change in bowel movements; any rash other than diaper rash. The latter, if severe, may also need medical treatment.

You know your baby better than anyone else. Trust your judgment and check with the baby's care-giver whenever you're concerned that some symptom or condition may be serious.

Clothes and Blankets for the Baby

Avoid making your baby too warm. Babies generally feel most comfortable in a room temperature around 68° to 70°. Comfortable indoor clothes would be just a shirt and diaper (or just a diaper when the weather's hot). When needed for more warmth indoors, add an outer garment such as a nightgown, a sleeping bag, or a stretch suit.

Use waterproof plastic pants over cloth diapers only for short periods of time, if at all. They can cause diaper rash by sealing in moisture. (They are not used with disposable diapers.)

For outdoor jaunts in colder weather, put on a stretch suit, a sweater, a hat, and possibly a snowsuit or pram suit. You might also put one or more blankets over the baby if it is to be carried in your arms or in a stroller or carriage.

When the baby is sleeping, cover it with a cotton receiving blanket or other light coverlet in mild weather, and with warmer blankets in cool weather. In the first few weeks, your baby may feel more secure when sleeping if it is wrapped rather snugly in a receiving blanket, laid on its side, and propped with a pillow or rolled-up blanket against its back. Being wrapped like this resembles the snugness of the womb, and babies appear to like it. They also seem to be annoyed by not being able to control random movements when more loosely wrapped. Their own movements sometimes evoke the startle reflex.

IV

Birth with Special Problems

16

⌒‿ᗡᘓ‿⌒

Selected Disorders of Childbearing

In a relatively few births of those predicted to be normal, complications may develop during or after labor and birth. Here's what you might need to know about the more common of these possibilities in order to reach intelligent decisions with the help of your care-giver.

Preterm Labor

Women start into labor before their fetuses are fully developed in less than 1 out of every 10 pregnancies that continue beyond about twenty weeks (or halfway through a full-term pregnancy). Infants are defined as premature if they are born before the thirty-seventh week of pregnancy or if they weigh less than 5½ pounds (2,500 grams) at birth.

A number of impressively effective techniques have been developed in recent years to help premature infants survive and grow normally. They are practiced by physicians expert in two new fields: *perinatology,* a subspecialty of obstetrics concentrating on health care for the fetus and the mother; and *neonatology,* a subspecialty of pediatrics concentrating on health care for the newborn.

Perinatologists and neonatologists typically practice in large hospitals, those classified as providing tertiary, or "Level III," care—care using technologic methods of the highest level. These hospitals, sometimes also called perinatal and/or neonatal centers, have neonatal intensive care units. In addition, however, perinatologists and neonatologists are also increasingly found in Level II institutions.

Risks and mortality rates are still relatively high, especially with the smaller premature infants.

Signs Indicating Preterm Labor

No generally accepted explanation of the causes of preterm labor has been developed. However, analyses have indicated that women with the following characteristics tend to go into preterm labor more often than other women:

- multiple fetus pregnancy (twins, triplets, etc.);
- preterm labor in a previous pregnancy (or a previous miscarriage in the second trimester);
- age under 18 or over 40;
- inflammation of the pelvis and kidneys;
- heavy smoking or chemical addiction;
- inadequate nutrition;
- exposure to diethylstilbestrol when you were a fetus;
- heavy psychological or physical stress;
- inadequate or absent prenatal care and supervision; or
- one of two other complications: toxemia (or pre-eclampsia) and placental abnormalities are complications which often lead to preterm birth.

Helping to Prevent Preterm Labor

Should any of the first eight conditions apply to you, you can take these steps to help prevent going into preterm labor (as recommended by the American College of Obstetricians and Gynecologists):

- Empty your bladder and bowel regularly and without delay, since prolonged retention of wastes increases the chances of pelvic infections.
- Avoid standing for long periods of time. In this way you will reduce congestion in your lower abdominal organs and thereby also lessen chances of infection.
- Avoid sexual intercourse and douching if your cervix has begun to thin and open early.

- Correct poor posture, and don't strain your lower back by inadvisable lifting. Over a long period of time, this may tire and weaken your pelvic organs.
- Ensure good nutrition.
- Reduce stress.

Stopping Preterm Labor if It Starts

In cases when labor does start prematurely despite efforts to avoid it, the woman should promptly inform her care-giver and follow the care-giver's advice carefully. Lying down and resting is often the first step recommended. Rest actually stops premature labor in something like half of all cases.

Women whose signs of premature labor persist are usually sent to the hospital for rest, observation, and possible medication to inhibit uterine activity and to relax the muscles of the uterus. The one medication currently approved by the Food and Drug Administration for use in stopping preterm labor after the nineteenth week of pregnancy is ritodrine. Ritodrine has side effects that increase in severity with the dosage; they can include stomach upset, heart palpitations, and increased glucose levels in the mother, all of which affect fetal well-being.

Studies of possible after-effects on infants whose mothers took ritodrine have indicated no detectable defects in growth and development up to age 2, which is as far as the studies have gone. Women who are advised to take it should discuss the risks in their specific situation with their care-givers.

If hospital bed rest, and possibly medication, succeed in arresting the preterm labor, the woman is often kept under observation for another day or two and then sent home to gradually resume normal activities.

Toxemia

Toxemia is a complication of pregnancy that may require taking steps to bring about preterm delivery. Its symptoms are divided by severity and are called pre-eclampsia and eclampsia. Pre-eclampsia is marked primarily by three symptoms, all of which are checked for at each prenatal visit:

- High blood pressure.

- Pronounced edema (retention of water in the tissues) evidenced by swelling, particularly in the hands and face and/or a sudden substantial weight gain. (Swelling in the feet frequently occurs in later pregnancy; it does not in itself indicate pre-eclampsia unless it appears with the other symptoms.)
- Protein in the form of albumin in the urine.

A fourth indication of more severe toxemia is disturbance or erratic functioning in the mother's vision.

Symptoms of eclampsia are convulsions and coma. They require immediate treatment.

Toxemia is serious enough to justify induced preterm labor or preterm delivery by cesarean section if indications show that it has advanced so far that the life of the fetus is endangered. Its advance from pre-eclampsia to eclampsia can also endanger the mother.

Safeguarding Actions

Sound prenatal care, and good prenatal nutrition especially, will prevent pre-eclampsia in the majority of cases. Other actions taken by expectant parents to guard against it include:

- Getting blood-pressure readings at regular prenatal checkups. (As a matter of course, readings under 140/90 are viewed as normal, though the individual's usual readings are taken into account.)
- Testing urine at prenatal checkups for any concentration of albumin.
- Seeking advice promptly should fluid retention bring fairly sudden and substantial increases in swelling in such areas as the ankles, fingers, wrists, and face. A sudden and substantial gain in weight may also indicate an increase in fluid retention signaling pre-eclampsia.
- Reporting promptly any irregularities in vision.

Correctives for Mild Pre-Eclampsia

If mild pre-eclampsia is found, two measures are usually advised: resting at frequent intervals, preferably lying on the left side since this takes the weight of the uterus off the vena cava (the large vein which returns circulation from the legs and lower trunk to the heart), or even bed rest much or all of the time; and careful attention to the diet to be sure that minerals and nutrients are in good balance.

Further Measures

Should high blood pressure, swelling, and other symptoms of toxemia worsen despite preventive measures, the expectant mother is hospitalized. Complete bed rest and sedation in the hospital often suffice to stabilize or reduce the symptoms—particularly high blood pressure. Failing that, medications to reduce blood pressure may be used.

Such measures aim at prolonging the pregnancy to term so long as fetal distress does not develop. But should serious fetal distress be evidenced (by such signs as slower heartbeat or activity, or meconium in the amniotic fluid) the baby would be delivered as soon as possible. The risks of preterm birth would then be less than the risks of toxemia.

Birth of premature infants would be carried out by either induced labor or cesarean section, depending on whether the fetus is judged to be less critically or more critically distressed (and also depending on the condition of the mother). It is felt that fetuses of under 3¼ pounds do not tolerate well the stress of labor.

DES Exposure

From the 1950s to about 1970, obstetricians widely prescribed DES (diethylstilbestrol) for pregnant women whose condition indicated a high risk of early miscarriage. Some of the daughters of those mothers who had taken DES in the first four months of pregnancy were found years later to have developed abnormalities of the vagina, cervix, and uterus. One such abnormality was a rare form of vaginal cancer (often easily curable when caught early). Another consisted of defects in the cervix, making it possibly too weak to support the weight of a pregnancy.

Estimates place the number of such DES-exposed daughters in the U.S. at about 3 million. Should you know that your mother was prescribed DES and wonder if it may have thus affected your genital organs, a simple doctor's office examination can sometimes but not always determine whether it did or did not.

Abruption

Premature labor can also result from a too-early separation of the placenta from the uterine wall, called *abruptio placentae*. It occurs rarely, in only about 1 in every 500 births. Formation of a blood clot behind the placenta is generally thought to cause the separation. It can also be related to a short umbilical cord, high blood pressure, or toxemia.

Bleeding flows from the area of the separation. This may appear as vaginal bleeding, or may be closed off in the upper uterus by the amniotic sac. Closed-off bleeding from abruptio placentae brings pain as the buildup of blood causes pressure inside the uterus. Such internal bleeding may be detected by a tenderness of the abdomen to the touch, coupled with increasing hardness. Concealed bleeding of this kind may also be detected by ultrasound techniques. In time, the blood loss may put the mother in shock.

Continued bleeding leads to fetal distress, with changes in the heart rate as the fetus gets less and less oxygen. Delivery in a case like this is usually done rapidly and by cesarean section.

In most instances when it does arise, *abruptio placentae* develops after the sixth month of pregnancy. *Any bleeding in pregnancy should be reported immediately to your care-provider.*

Respiratory Distress Syndrome

Respiratory distress syndrome—called RDS—represents a leading cause of mortality among premature infants. It is a condition found in fetuses born so early that the insides of the air sacs in their lungs have not yet developed a coating of substances called surfactants. Surfactants keep the sides of the air sacs from sticking together when the baby exhales. They prevent partial or full collapse of the air sacs and lungs and possible asphyxiation.

Laboratory tests for the relative amounts of two chemicals in the woman's amniotic fluid can help determine what risk of RDS a fetus will run if born prematurely. The tests are valuable in deciding whether the fetus has enough surfactant to survive if delivered immediately, or whether every effort should instead be made to continue the pregnancy and delay delivery despite risks to the fetus or the mother due to other conditions.

This type of laboratory analysis is called the L/S ratio test, because it establishes the ratio between lecithin and sphingomyelin, two chemicals in the amniotic fluid. Ratios of at least twice as much "L" as "S" (expressed in such figures as 2.2 to 1 or 2.5 to 1) indicate with about 97 percent certainty that the fetus will not develop RDS, so that prompt birth should be safe.

L/S ratios of at least 3.0 to 1 are advised for safety from RDS if the woman has diabetes or if certain other rare conditions are present (such as incompatibility in blood types between mother and fetus). Presence of meconium in the amniotic fluid (as evidenced by greenish or brownish feces of the fetus in the fluid) may make L/S ratio findings unreliable, and may itself be an indication of fetal distress.

Amniotic fluid for the test is usually obtained by amniocentesis.

RDS has sometimes appeared in infants delivered by induced labor or by cesarean section carried out at times arbitrarily set for reasons of convenience (rather than as an emergency)—especially in situations in which the due date was not known with reasonable certainty. Tests for L/S ratio are particularly important in order to avoid cases like this.

After the thirty-fifth week of pregnancy another test, which detects the presence of an additional chemical in the amniotic fluid, can provide still more conclusive findings on RDS hazards for a fetus. (The chemical is phosphatidylglycerol.)

Laboratory tests for RDS require several hours to produce results. Findings of RDS with lesser but reasonably high degrees of probability can be obtained in about thirty minutes with a third type of test, called the foam stability test, or shake test. It can be helpful on occasions in which the severely weakened condition of the fetus or the mother makes it vital to deliver the baby safely as soon as possible.

In this test, the care-giver puts a sample of amniotic fluid in a glass vessel, adds alcohol, seals the vessel, and shakes it hard. Foam forms around the edge of the surface of the liquid. If the foam remains without dissolving for fifteen minutes or more, there is only a very small chance that the fetus would develop RDS if delivered at that time.

Miscarriage

Spontaneous loss of the fetus through the vagina before the twenty-eighth week (or end of the seventh month) is popularly called miscarriage rather than premature birth. Professional terminology for loss of the fetus during pregnancy is as follows: "spontaneous abortion" loss before the twenty-first week; "immature labor" loss during the twenty-first through twenty-seventh week; and "preterm labor" loss during the twenty-eighth through the thirty-sixth week.

Miscarriages happen most often very early in pregnancy, and less and less often beyond the second and third months. (Ten to fifteen percent of pregnancies terminate in spontaneous abortion.) Fetuses expelled before the twenty-eighth week have difficulty surviving because they have not developed sufficiently for extrauterine life. However, because of developments in neonatal intensive care techniques, fetuses born very early are surviving in increasing numbers.

In general, sound prenatal care provides the best protection against miscarriage for persons who are physically normal. However, miscarriages often result from mere chance rather than anything the expectant parents and their care-givers can control. Such chance causes include an accidentally or genetically flawed egg or sperm cell; chance failure in other delicate processes, such as the implantation of the fertilized ovum in the uterine lining, or in the working of the placenta; and chance effects of a chronic health problem, such as diabetes, high blood pressure, or a thyroid condition.

But miscarriages may also result from factors that the individual can often do something about—by following a program of good prenatal care. Among those factors are infection, inadequate nutrition, a congenital weakness of the cervix, called an "incompetent cervix" (which can be resolved by early diagnosis and suturing until labor starts), and toxic substances in the home environment or workplace.

Precautions

Some women with chronic health conditions such as heart disease or diabetes may run higher than normal risks of miscarriage. What special risks you may run can be appraised in your early prenatal physical examinations (or even prepregnancy examinations). Your care-givers can then advise you on the precautions most likely to prevent miscarriage.

Vaginal spotting or bleeding may be an early sign of approaching miscarriage, but many women who spot or bleed in the early months continue on to perfectly normal, healthy births. *Tell your care-giver promptly if you have such bleeding.* He or she might advise you to avoid as much strain and fatigue as you can, check your nutrition and eating, and perhaps suspend intercourse until two weeks or more after the bleeding stops.

If You Have a Miscarriage

Unavoidable miscarriage takes place when you have substantial bleeding with the passage of clots, along with a regular series of cramps that can start up and stop two or more times. (In addition, examination by a care-giver may show that your cervix has dilated.)

Though it can be very hard to do, try to save the discharge of a miscarriage in a glass jar or plastic container. This may be helpful to specialists in deciding whether you have expelled everything, and may eliminate the need for special medical treatment.

Passage of the embryo (or fetus) and the entire placenta is termed a complete miscarriage. Incomplete miscarriages are ones in which some or all of the products of conception are left inside the uterus. Their incidence is higher from about the tenth week through the twentieth week than at other times of pregnancy.

If you've had an incomplete loss, and bleeding and cramps go on for more than a few days, immediately see your care-giver. It may be necessary to remove the remaining tissues by a treatment called a dilation and curettage (D and C), which involves scraping the uterine lining while you're anesthetized.

Afterward, you will usually be advised to wait a few months before your next conception. During this period you may go through a mourning process similar to that after any personal loss. This is normal and healthy. Talk over your feelings with your partner or other loved ones.

Ectopic or Tubal Pregnancy

In rare instances, the fertilized ovum implants in one of the fallopian tubes or, very rarely, in other abdominal tissue not within the uterus. Such implantation begins what is termed an ectopic pregnancy. These occur at rates varying from 1 in every 300 to 1 in every 80 pregnancies, as reflected in the records of various hospitals. In 95 out of 100 ectopic pregnancies, the ovum implants in one of the fallopian tubes, hence the term tubal pregnancy.

Tubal pregnancies tend to result in most cases from a prior infection of the tubes, scarring from past surgery, or congenital tube abnormalities so that the fertilized ovum encounters a barrier as it travels toward the uterine cavity. They are often evidenced by such signs as:

- a missed period;
- appearance of some of the bodily changes of early pregnancy (but not in all cases of tubal pregnancy);
- a week or more after the missed period, repeated sensations of a slight, passing pain in the side (which often goes unnoticed at the time);
- about two to four weeks after the missed period, a limited amount of reddish brown vaginal discharge or spotting.

Bleeding from the uterus and pain in the abdomen are the main signs of a tubal pregnancy. Women experiencing them should tell their care-provider promptly. A tubal pregnancy can result in sudden, very intense abdominal pain when the tube ruptures. Internal hemorrhage may be causing the pain. Ectopic pregnancy requires surgical treatment. Transfusion may be required if internal hemorrhage has occurred.

Having had one ectopic pregnancy does not preclude the possibility of a later normal pregnancy and birth. Studies indicate that, after a tubal pregnancy, half or more of later pregnancies resulted in live births. However, some women may have another ectopic experience.

Hydramnios

About 1 liter of amniotic fluid—slightly more than a quart—normally surrounds the fetus in the later months of pregnancy. The presence of 2 liters or more of fluid is defined as hydramnios (or polyhydramnios), an abnormal condition of excess fluid.

Pregnancies in which there is a small amount of excess fluid are not uncommon, and they result in no discomfort or other difficulty. In only about 1 in every 1,000 or more pregnancies does severe hydramnios appear, in which 3 or more liters of fluid develop. This can be a sign of fetal abnormalities requiring diagnostic sonography. With that much excess fluid, women experience difficulties resulting from the overdistension of the uterus.

An opposite condition of far too little amniotic fluid (called oligohydramnios) develops in a very small number of cases. Your care-giver should easily be able to diagnose and advise you about the condition when you get a checkup.

Breech or Other Nonvertex Presentation

Only some 3 in every 100 unborn infants settle into a buttocks-down, head-up position in the uterus—called a breech presentation—shortly before the due date and labor. Possible risks to the baby in vaginal birth are increased with the breech position. As a result, most care-givers recommend that women with babies in breech presentations go to the hospital for birth and advise against trying to give birth in a birth center or in a planned home birth.

External Version

Some practitioners may gently try to turn the fetus to a head-down position after about the thirtieth week of pregnancy. They have the pregnant woman lie on her back and relax, and then they carefully see if they can push the fetus around from the outside of the woman's abdomen. External version should be tried only by someone skilled at it, and only when the woman is not anesthetized and is alert to report any discomfort or pain she feels in the process.

In considering version, you might observe two guidelines suggested by experience:

- Start discussing external version with your care-provider before your thirtieth week of pregnancy, and have it attempted before your thirty-second week. Other practitioners favor a later time because breech babies sometimes turn to a normal position shortly before labor.

- It is important to find a practitioner in your locale who is skilled at external version. Ask your care-giver (or other sources, such as the teacher of your prenatal classes) to suggest a practitioner experienced in performing successful versions.

Cesareans for Breech Babies

In the course of vaginal delivery of a breech baby, complications can develop, including a pinched cord or other severe oxygen deprivation. Care-providers accordingly advise that vaginal delivery should be attempted only if indications for success look especially favorable. Among such indications are a large enough opening between the woman's pelvic bones and a baby weighing less than about 8 pounds, which together indicate that the baby's head is likely to be able to pass easily through the pelvic opening. If these indications are not adequate, or if there is other evidence of problems with a vaginal birth, the practitioner will recommend birth by cesarean section.

Because of the growing trend toward the use of cesarean delivery for all breech presentations, some obstetricians have not had the opportunity to finely hone their skills and may feel reluctant to attempt a vaginal birth in a case of breech presentation.

Transverse Presentation

In much rarer instances—only 1 in every 200 to 400 pregnancies—the fetus has settled into a sideways, or transverse, position in the uterus just before labor. Care-givers always recommend going to a hospital for labor and delivery in such cases.

Sometimes a transverse fetus shifts to a head-down position very early in labor. If it does not, the care-giver may attempt external version, stopping if monitors detect fetal distress or if the woman feels pain. Unless the position of the fetus shifts or can be shifted, care-givers will recommend cesarean section for delivery.

Abnormal Labor Patterns

Prolonged Latent Phase

The long phase of first-stage labor in which the cervix slowly becomes completely effaced and starts opening is called the latent phase. Its ending is marked by the start of the active phase, which brings relatively rapid dilation with stronger contractions coming faster, at three-minute and two-minute intervals.

Latent-phase labor normally runs up to ten or twelve hours for a woman having a first baby (a primigravida or nullipara), or up to about six or eight hours for a woman having a baby after her first (multigravida).

Latent-phase labor will run longer in a small proportion of pregnancies. In some of these cases, the cervix remains rigid and thick despite normally regular and strong uterine contractions. In others, the contractions are weaker and less regular than normal and the cervix does not fully efface. Such unusually long early labor is termed prodromal labor.

Treatment for prodromal labor usually consists first in simply waiting beyond the customarily defined time spans of latent-phase labor if the woman is not too tired. With some women and pregnancies, the latent phase naturally runs longer than usual. However, if the woman grows exhausted after fifteen hours or more of labor, treatment may call for injection of a sedative to give her and her uterus rest for about an eight-hour period.

More than 8 out of 10 women treated in this way went on, after the rest, to normal active-phase labor in one group studied. Almost all of the remaining women in the group later went into active labor after being given oxytocin to stimulate the uterus. The very small proportion who did not went on to deliveries by cesarean section.

Delay in Labor

In other cases representing small proportions of pregnancies, labor does not unfold normally in other respects.

In a few of these cases, the fetus does not descend (or does not descend far enough) into the pelvis. Such an occurrence is usually judged to be an instance of "cephalopelvic disproportion"—too large a diameter of the baby's head, or too small an opening in the mother's pelvic bone, for easy passage of the baby.

Such stoppages or "arrests" in the process of labor and birth almost always leave no alternative but a trial with chemical stimulation in a hospital setting, and if effective labor does not result, delivery by cesarean section. The reason customarily given in medical records for cesareans of this kind is "failure to progress" in labor. If this term should be applied to you, it simply means a delay in labor. In no way does it imply any failure on your part as a mother.

Other Unexpected Developments

Placenta Previa

In less than 1 in 200 pregnancies, the fertilized ovum implants relatively low in the uterus, causing the placenta to partly or fully cover the top of the cervix inside the uterus. Called placenta previa, this condition develops by chance, many research specialists think. The difficulty becomes apparent as the cervix "ripens" in preparation for birth. As it thins and opens, the placental surface is exposed, permitting blood to escape.

Painless vaginal bleeding is both the sign and major hazard of placenta previa. Bleeding usually starts after the seventh month with spotting or a small single discharge of bright red blood. After a few days or another week or two the bleeding starts recurring regularly, becoming more heavy as time goes on. In rare cases the woman may go on into late pregnancy or even labor without showing any sign of having a placenta previa.

Practitioners advise against any vaginal examination if the bleeding is light and the due date is only a few weeks away. Vaginal examination might increase bleeding.

Ultrasound scans or sonograms are often advised since they represent the surest means of determining the location of the placenta (and hence its potential risk for placenta previa) with minimal or no harm.

Following a diagnosis of previa, vaginal examination in a hospital is customarily made if delivery is expected right away or if the due date has arrived. At the examination, standby preparations are made, including preparations for possible whole-blood transfusion and cesarean section.

Complications with the Umbilical Cord

Looped cord: Umbilical cords of normal lengths are long enough (35 to 70 centimeters, or 15 to 30 inches) to permit considerable free movement of the fetus. Thus it is possible for the cord to become looped one or more times around the neck, arm, leg, or other parts of the body. A nuchal cord (around the neck) is not uncommon at birth. Usually it is loose and can be slipped back over the baby's body or brought forward over its head, but if not, it can be clamped, cut, and unwound before the birth continues.

The cord poses no difficulty in labor unless its specific position causes it to be compressed, reducing oxygen supplied to the fetus (and resulting in an oxygen-deprived condition called fetal hypoxia).

In rare instances of severe compression with signs of fetal distress recognizable to an experienced practitioner, delivery by cesarean section is necessary.

Short cord: Only in very rare cases is the cord markedly shorter than the average length of 21 or 22 inches. If the cord is extremely short, the fetus may evidence serious distress as the cord is stretched during descent in labor and the vital blood vessels in the cord are narrowed by the stretching. Cesarean deliveries are required in such cases.

Prolapsed cord: In about 1 in every 200 labors, when the fetal presenting part has not become fixed (engaged) in the pelvis or when a bend or loop of the umbilical cord becomes positioned in the lower part of the uterus, the cord gets squeezed between the fetal body and the uterine wall (occult prolapse). It can wash through the cervix at the time the amniotic membranes rupture. It is in large part for this reason that you are urged to report promptly any suspected rupture of your membranes to your care-giver.

The cord loop may even extend through the cervix and appear at the vaginal outlet. This condition is termed complete prolapse of the cord. Take these two emergency actions immediately should it develop:

1. Assume a knee-chest position in which you rest your body on your knees with hips high and your chest down on the level of your knees, with your head lying on your folded arms. This may move the fetus off the cord and permit free circulation to continue.
2. Get to the nearest hospital as fast as possible (while maintaining the knee-chest position on a stretcher or other flat surface, if you can).

A prolapsed cord represents a very serious condition for the baby because the presenting part can partly or completely compress the cord and cut off its own oxygen supply.

A cord that will prolapse cannot be detected before labor begins. Failure of the presenting part to engage in the pelvis may indicate the condition. Once the cervix has dilated—and if the amniotic membranes have not yet ruptured—vaginal examination may identify a "forelying" cord. It may be felt inside the intact membranes beside the baby's body in the lower part of the uterus. Diagnosis of a forelying cord—a potentially prolapsed cord—early in labor usually leads to a recommendation of delivery by cesarean section.

Infant mortality runs high among cases of prolapsed cord. The condition poses essentially no danger to the mother, however.

There is no known method for preventing prolapsed cord, other than not performing amniotomy (artificial rupture of the membranes) unless the presenting part is well fixed in the pelvis (thus blocking descent of the cord).

Rh Incompatibility

In order to avoid a possible future complication that could be very serious, one simple precaution should be taken by any expectant mother who has blood of the Rh-negative type, if the baby's father has blood of the far more common Rh-positive type. That precaution is to have an intramuscular injection of Rh-immune globulin in about the twenty-eighth to thirtieth week of pregnancy (a timing now recommended by the American College of Obstetricians and Gynecologists). Becoming immunized in this way keeps the woman's system from making antibodies to any Rh-positive cells that may enter her blood from the fetus.

It's important to prevent formation of such antibodies, for they will remain permanently in the woman's system. In later pregnancies they can pass through the placenta into the fetus, and then destroy its Rh-positive red blood cells. Fetal heart failure, anemia, and death can occur as a result.

Other Complications

A number of other complications can arise, but these either are very rare—with an incidence lower than 1 out of 1,000 pregnancies—or they generally cannot be diagnosed or prevented in advance. A thoroughly capable care-giver together with a system of good, comprehensive prenatal care represents your best means for either avoiding them or dealing with them effectively should they occur.

17

Cesarean Birth and Vaginal Birth with Instruments

During your pregnancy or labor, you might be told that you need one or the other of two types of operative procedures: cesarean birth (with delivery of the baby through incisions in the abdomen after the mother has been anesthetized), or vaginal birth with instruments (in which obstetrical forceps or a vacuum extractor is used to help draw the baby through the birth canal).

Both types of birth are referred to as "operative obstetrics," even though the latter consists of assisting a natural process with instruments rather than an "operation" involving incisions.

Many expectant parents leave decisions about these types of birth completely up to the professionals providing their maternity care. They believe that long professional training and experience are needed in order to decide when and how these births should be carried out.

However, decisions about even these types of births remain your responsibility. Legally, they cannot be attempted without your informed consent (unless your situation becomes a life-threatening emergency for you or your baby). And increasing numbers of expectant parents and authorities on childbearing point out that a number of basic features of such births can in fact be decided by the parents, with the help of cooperative care-givers (especially if those features are talked over in advance, during pregnancy). Making these decisions with professional help can give many parents a more satisfying birth experience, in much the same way as for a vaginal birth without instruments.

283

Vaginal Birth with Instruments

Forceps-Assisted Deliveries

Limitation on the use of forceps in a vaginal birth is a matter about which you should decide after discussions with your care-giver (or with prospective care-givers).

In essence, forceps are instruments with two thin curved blades that fit on the head of the fetus. When used to assist breech birth, forceps grip the infant's "after-coming" head.

Forceps should be used only with the mother fully relaxed under general or local anesthesia, for the thin blades can accidentally bruise or tear her tissues if resistance is encountered. In using them, the physician inserts the blades one at a time through the vagina, positions them on the infant's head, and holds them in place. The handles protrude from the vagina. The physician then pulls on the handles to draw the fetus down the birth canal, or turns the handles to rotate the baby into a more beneficial position and then pulls.

Forceps can safely be employed for only a few types of problems in labor today. Most problems that occasioned the use of forceps in past eras can be far more safely handled by modern techniques for vaginal deliveries (such as stimulation of the uterus with oxytocin in the case of protracted labor), or by cesarean delivery.

The careful use of forceps can be justified at present in these situations:

- Clear evidence of severe fetal distress developing when the woman has not yet completed the second stage of labor, but when the baby is well down in the birth canal.

- Clearly demonstrated inability of the woman to push out the baby after having been in second-stage labor well over two hours for a first birth or more than one hour for a birth after the first. Sometimes called "second-stage lack of progress of labor," this condition may be caused by various factors, including near-exhaustion of the woman, epidural anesthesia, weak contractions or weak abdominal muscles, pelvic-floor tissues unusually resistant to stretching around the baby's head, unusually large size of the baby, and baby's head facing the side or front of the pelvis.

- Imminently life-threatening complications developing in second-stage labor, such as a severe abruptio placentae, in which the baby's life would be lost if forceps were not applied.

- Need for the woman to avoid hard pushing during second-stage labor for such compelling reasons as a heart condition so serious that

284

the mother and baby would be endangered if she pushed strenuously, or a rare eye condition in which the mother must avoid building up pressure because of a risk of detached retina.

- With premature infants, to shorten the second stage of labor and reduce pressure on the immature fetal head.

The basic rule to follow on forceps is, accordingly:

Ask that forceps not be used, except when

(1) ONE OF THE ABOVE CONDITIONS APPLIES, AND

(2) THE BABY'S SCALP CAN BE SEEN AT THE VAGINAL OPENING WITH EACH CONTRACTION.

Use of forceps when the baby's scalp can be seen readily at the vaginal outlet represents what is called a low-forceps delivery. Little risk to the baby and the mother is posed in this case (generally less than with a cesarean attempted at a similar point in labor, for instance). In mid-forceps use, the fetal head is engaged in the pelvis but has not reached the pelvic floor. High forceps refers to a situation in which the fetal head is not yet engaged in the pelvis.

Mid-forceps deliveries pose greater hazards to the baby and mother than low-forceps deliveries. High-forceps deliveries pose such a high risk of serious injury that in general they are contraindicated. Cesarean section is preferable to a mid-forceps or high-forceps delivery.

Major additional conditions that should be met if at all possible before carrying out a low-forceps delivery include:

- The amniotic sac membranes are ruptured.
- Bladder of the woman must have been drained by a catheter to keep it from being injured.
- Bony pelvis must be large enough and baby's head must be small enough for the baby to pass through the opening without injury.
- Anesthesia must be given to the woman and the anesthesiologist must stand by for immediate further action if needed.

Talk over your preferences concerning forceps with your care-giver (or prospective care-givers) as early as possible in your pregnancy. Reach a full understanding on your concerns regarding any possible need for forceps use that may arise. Add those mutually-arrived-at decisions to your statement of preferences for your scheduled or backup hospital.

Keep in mind that the use of forceps has declined in recent years and that younger practitioners may not be skilled in their use. Nurse-midwives are not educated to use forceps.

Vacuum Extractors

The vacuum extractor is an instrument designed to be used instead of forceps in situations for which low-forceps and mid-forceps deliveries are appropriate. Few practitioners use vacuum extractors in the United States; they are more widely employed in Europe.

Extractors consist of a convex plastic skull cap that fits over the rear (occiput) of the baby's head. Air is then drawn out to form a partial vacuum so that the baby's scalp is tightly gripped. The physician can then exert force to move the baby down the birth canal—much as with forceps but without the additional bulk that forceps provide.

Scrapes and cuts in the baby's scalp can result from use of the extractor. It can also cause blood clotting under the scalp. Occasional internal bleeding within the fetal skull or eyes, and even a few fetal deaths, have been reported as consequences.

Three advantages claimed for the vacuum extractor are that (1) the woman's cervix need not be fully dilated in order for its use to be attempted, (2) it does not result in injuries to the mother and baby as serious or as frequent as possible injuries from the use of forceps, and (3) anesthesia is not necessary, a feature that can avoid risks to the fetus in a case of fetal distress.

Should your physician care-giver happen to be experienced in using the vacuum extractor, discuss in advance the precautions he or she will take to avoid any possible injury in using it in your labor should the need arise. Mutually decide on those precautions that are important to you, and include them in your consent form preferences at the hospital.

Use of forceps and vacuum extractors has been defined as inappropriate in freestanding birth centers, by both the American Public Health Association and the National Association of Childbearing Centers.

Cesarean Births

Increasing numbers of parents having cesareans want their birth experience to include one or more of the features of family-centered childbirth such as:

- Having the mother fully conscious and aware through the use of regional, often epidural, rather than general anesthesia.
- Having the father (or other support partner) stay with the mother through labor and birth as well as postoperative recovery, while actively giving the mother emotional support, encouragement, affection, reassurance, and companionship.
- Having the newborn baby start bonding with its parents right after birth, and having some elements of a Leboyer "gentle birth."
- Having the baby stay with the mother in her hospital room rather than in the infant nursery after initial recovery from surgery and while she remains in the hospital.
- Having the mother breastfeed if she so chooses.
- Having the father visit or stay with the mother and baby in the hospital through special daylong and evening visiting hours.
- Having any older sisters or brothers of the baby visit as soon after the birth as the mother feels up to it.

You should be able to arrange any such practices you want through careful selection of your care-givers and hospital (or the hospital backup to a birth center or home birth in case you may need a cesarean).

The High Rate of Cesareans

Rates at which physicians perform cesarean births have risen rapidly in recent years. One in every 5 or 6 pregnant women in America today experiences cesarean rather than vaginal birth. Fewer than 1 in every 20 had cesarean birth only a quarter-century ago.

Much of the increase came in the 1970s. Nationwide, the cesarean birth rate soared from 5.5 percent in 1970 to 15.2 percent in 1978. In 1983 20.3 percent of all deliveries were by cesarean section (according to preliminary national figures). Obstetrician Norbert Gleicher commented: "A review of underlying causes for these developments suggests that only a more efficient peer review process, involving individual physicians as well as institutions, will lead to a decline of unacceptably high cesarean section rates in this country." [1]

Although the increase in cesareans has in fact benefited the mothers and infants in a number of cases, most informed observers conclude that in cesareans some proportion of the increase is not sufficiently justified and even potentially harmful. For example, two such observers state that "reducing the number of cesareans has become a subject of intense interest among doctors, medical institutions, groups of concerned citizens, and governmental and professional agencies." They go on to emphasize: *"The consensus is that many cesareans can be safely avoided."* (Italics in the original.) [2]

The key points concerning cesareans are:

1. Take reasonable precautions to avoid running the risk of an unnecessary cesarean. (Cesareans present 2 to 4 times the risk of maternal mortality as compared to vaginal birth, according to the National Institutes of Health.)
2. Plan in advance for the practices you would want in a possible cesarean, just in case one may prove necessary in your case.
3. If you do need a cesarean birth, try to feel just as positive about it and your baby as you would with a vaginal birth, for the emotional and physical well-being of the baby, yourself, and your partner.

Avoiding an Unnecessary Cesarean

According to the NIH,[3] the reasons for performing a cesarean have in recent years in the U.S. broken down as follows:

Reason	Percentage of All Cesareans
Dystocia (failure to progress, cephalo-pelvic disproportion, fetal size, abnormal fetal position other than breech)	31%
Repeat cesarean	31%
Breech position of fetus	12%
Fetal distress	5%
Other (largely chronic condition)	21%

From this you can see that you would probably not know of a clear-cut need for a cesarean early in your pregnancy. Care-givers can determine such a need at the outset of pregnancy only under two conditions: repeat cesareans and certain chronic conditions.

The American College of Obstetricians and Gynecologists now recommends that a subsequent cesarean is necessary only if the previous one was performed for one of the chronic health problems indicated on page 289 (which is likely to recur), or if the previous incision in the uterus was not a "transverse low segment section," a horizontal incision. And in fact, the number of mandatory repeat cesareans being performed today is far smaller than the 31 percent indicated for the recent years covered by the table.

A few chronic illnesses or congenital physical conditions call for a cesarean delivery. Among these are diabetes mellitus, high blood pressure, and heart disease, if they are severe enough to result in danger to either the fetus or the mother. Among other very rare conditions are abnormal growths (such as tumors and fibroids) in the uterus that require or had earlier required incisions through the wall of the uterus. (Diabetic women are now increasingly being brought to term for vaginal birth, thanks to recently improved techniques for supervised self-monitoring of blood-sugar levels with insulin adjustment.)

These reasons for a cesarean are forseeable long in advance, and are included in the "Other" in the table. They account for much less than the full 21 percent of cesarean deliveries carried out for all reasons in the "Other" category. A very rare additional reason among those in this "Other" category is pregnancy with triplets or a larger multiple birth. (Triplets occur naturally in less than 1 in every 7,500 pregnancies, and quadruplets or larger multiple births far less often; multiple-birth incidence rises particularly among women given fertility drugs or medications to stimulate ovulation.)

The remaining reasons in the table arise only very late in pregnancy or in labor. For instance:

- prolonged labor (often called failure to progress),
- cephalo-pelvic disproportion (too large a fetal head for the mother's pelvic opening) of a type that can be ascertained only during labor,
- fetal size generally too large for the pelvis opening, and
- abnormal nonbreech presentation of the fetus (a side-lying presentation rather than the normal head or breech-down presentation for birth).

Breech presentation of the fetus as another possible reason for cesarean birth cannot be determined with certainty until late pregnancy. These babies sometimes spontaneously shift to a head-down presentation in the last few days before labor begins. They may also be rotated by external version before labor starts, as described in Chapter 16.

Cesareans are very widely recommended, though, once the breech presentation is definite at the onset of labor. Nationally, more than 60 percent of all breech babies are delivered by cesarean section, according to the NIH.[4] However, vaginal birth "should remain an acceptable obstetrical choice" for breech babies, they recommend, under the following conditions:

- expected weight at birth of less than 8 but more than 5½ pounds,
- mother's pelvis is of normal size and form,

- "frank" breech presentation without a "hyperextended" head (this presentation involves fewer complications than other types), and
- delivery by a physician experienced in vaginal breech births.

Fetal distress, a condition of the fetus caused by a substantial reduction in its supply of oxygen-laden blood, represents the reason for only 1 in every 20 cesareans. Its appearance before late pregnancy is thought to be very rare in normally healthy women. In the case of most cesareans done because of fetal distress, the distress has been recognized during labor.

Much controversy surrounds the use of fetal distress as a reason for cesarean births. On the one hand, critics charge that physicians too often hastily, mistakenly, and defensively rely on the indications of electronic fetal monitoring (EFM) to carry out cesareans. For example, one study of the especially careful use of EFM at the hospital of the medical school of the University of California at Davis concluded that the type of EFM finding "classically thought to indicate fetal distress was wrong about 75 percent of the time." [5] Those misleading EFM indications had resulted in cesareans for assumed fetal distress.

On the other hand, defenders reply to the critics by arguing that physicians who rely on EFM indications of fetal distress perform cesareans in order to prevent brain damage or other birth defects that might be caused by oxygen deprivation in labor.

Arbiters agree that many babies delivered by cesareans because EFM had indicated fetal distress show no evidence after birth of actually having been in such distress—mainly in view of the fact that their Apgar scores are high to very high. These arbiters therefore often urge more careful and informed use of EFM rather than its elimination.

More dependable decisions will result if indications of fetal distress from EFM are confirmed by a fetal-scalp blood-sample test, some arbiters point out. One comparative study of groups of electronically monitored women showed a drop of six percentage points in the number of cesareans when scalp sampling was used (from 18 to 12 percent).[6]

Before making the test, the mother's cervix must have dilated to about 2 centimeters or more and her amniotic sac must have ruptured. The test is carried out by obtaining a drop or two of fetal blood after making a slight scalp incision through the dilated cervix. Immediate lab analysis of the blood sample indicates whether or not the fetus has serious oxygen deprivation, or hypoxia.

One drawback is the need for twenty-four-hour laboratory capability. Also, additional examinations during labor with the membranes ruptured expose both mother and fetus to infection.

Choosing a Care-Giver

Learning as much as you reasonably can about your own condition and indications for a cesarean can certainly help you and your care-giver make informed decisions on management of your labor and birth. One of the most efficient and effective ways of learning is through discussions with a care-giver who has:

- a personal commitment to vaginal birth and avoidance of a cesarean delivery if at all possible;

- expert and up-to-date knowledge, through high-quality education and experience in attending childbearing women plus continuing work to keep informed of current developments;

- the willingness and ability to answer any questions or concerns you may have, giving full, unbiased explanations and information to your complete satisfaction;

- a professional orientation including respect and willingness to cooperate with you regarding your preferences on basic features of your pregnancy and birth experience.

You can ask these specific questions to help ascertain a care-giver's commitment to avoiding unnecessary cesareans:

What cesarean rate do you have in your maternity practice? For individuals and hospitals, below 10 percent is impressively low, from 10 to 14 percent reflects some special effort to avoid needless cesareans, and 15 percent or above reflects less commitment to avoiding cesareans. (These figures are approximate guidelines.)

What is the cesarean rate at the hospital you'll use for my labor and delivery (or the hospital you'll use for backup if labor and delivery will take place at a birth center or at home)? The guidelines are given in the question above.

Does that hospital require second opinions or peer reviews for each cesarean done there? Second opinions are obtained from a senior professional before each cesarean; peer reviews are made after the cesareans, on a weekly or monthly basis. Requiring either type of appraisal probably reflects a commitment to appropriate use of cesarean birth.

You can also get helpful advice about the attitudes of specific caregivers in your locale by asking informed individuals—childbirth educators conducting your prenatal classes, classmates who have had babies recently, and members of local chapters of parenting organizations such as cesarean support groups.

If You Use a Practitioners' Group

If your care is provided by a group of practitioners rather than a specific individual, a few additional steps are necessary to ensure reasonable protection against a needless cesarean.

1. Ask if those qualities that are important to you are shared by all group members. Care-givers providing maternity care in a group are likely to hold much the same views, but ask the one or two members you talk with at the outset in order to get their assurance.
2. Try to get acquainted with all members of the group during your appointments for prenatal health care, to see if their views on possible cesareans are sympathetic to your preferences. You will also learn what the different members are like personally. This is important because you will receive care from whichever group member is available at the time you enter labor.
3. Be especially sure to have copies of a written statement of your preferences for labor and birth kept with your hospital chart after your admission. This precaution can prove useful if a group member less familiar with your preferences should attend you when labor starts.

Choosing a Hospital

Which hospital you go to (or may go to) for your labor and birth can significantly raise or lower your chances of having a cesarean delivery. Rates for cesarean deliveries as a percentage of all births vary widely among hospitals. For instance, in one large American city, cesarean rates were 9.2 percent at one hospital, 24 percent at another, and 36.7 percent at a third.

Variations like these do not result necessarily from serving different populations with varying risks. They often reflect differences in the way in which hospital staff members respond to labor and delivery. For example, two additional hospitals in the same city both serve essentially similar middle-class families, yet their cesarean rates were respectively 17.9 percent and 32.4 percent.

You might also ask the hospital about its infant and maternal loss rates. The type of mortality rate most meaningful for the hospital's handling of labor and birth is the neonatal mortality rate, the number of deaths of infants per 1,000 births through the first twenty-eight days of life. Other rates officially recorded include the perinatal mortality rate (deaths of fetuses or babies per 1,000 pregnancies from the end of the twenty-eighth week of pregnancy through the first twenty-eight days of life), the postneonatal mortality rate (deaths of babies from the twenty-ninth day through the first year of life), and the infant mortality rate (deaths from birth through the first year of life).

A hospital may be reluctant to provide such rates based on their impression that they are hard for laypersons to interpret correctly. If so, you might ask for those neonatal statistics together with the hospital's interpretation. Should the hospital still refuse, you might reasonably assume it would also be unwilling to cooperate with you in other ways.

Low-income mothers and mothers who have not received prenatal health care have infant loss rates that usually run about twice the rates of others. Therefore, when you ask for infant mortality rates you should also ask for the percentages of such mothers served.

Illustrated by the cases of three large hospitals in a suburban area, with each handling more than 1,500 births a year and serving some 10 percent low-income mothers; here's how those hospitals compared:

	Cesarean Rate %	Neonatal Mortality Rate % *
Hospital A	14.2%	5.5 per 1,000
Hospital B	23.2%	6.2 per 1,000
Hospital C	16.0%	7.6 per 1,000

As you can see, Hospital A is likely to be a sounder choice on the combined grounds of avoiding a needless cesarean and also reducing risks to the baby (other things being equal among the three hospitals).

Hospitals are often required to report statistics on their annual cesarean rates and maternal/neonatal mortality rates to the public health departments of their local and state governments. If necessary, you might obtain the figures through those public health offices.

Here are several other questions to ask any hospital you are considering:

• What protocols does the hospital have on cesareans? Protocols are written policy directives of the hospital concerning treatment of patients. They may indicate policies either requiring cesareans on the basis of arbitrarily fixed criteria, or allowing cesareans only if proven to be thoroughly justified after a number of precautionary

---

* See Appendix B. *How to Avoid a Cesarean Section,* by Christopher Norwood.

steps. Discuss the protocols with your care-giver to see if they would tend to raise or lower your chances of having an unnecessary cesarean at that hospital.

- Does the hospital use the fetal-scalp blood-sampling test as a further check on EFM diagnosis?
- Does the hospital permit you to provide a written statement of your preferences for treatment during labor and birth that will be kept with your chart at all times?

   You or your care-giver can write such a statement after you decide on your preferences for a vaginal birth or a cesarean birth (if the latter should be needed). Having the statement kept with your chart as a patient at the hospital will help make sure that your preferences will be honored, on the chance that your care-giver may be called away or delayed briefly during your labor.

   You might also ask if the hospital's maternity service includes certified nurse-midwives or special homelike birthing rooms. Even if you plan a type of birth that would not involve a CNM or a birthing room, their presence would be a general indication that the hospital has policies in support of normal vaginal birth.

Checking the Hospital's Facilities

Because of the increased possibility of cesarean birth today, you must be sure that the hospital you choose will be safe for a cesarean should you need one. This applies equally to a hospital that represents your first choice for the setting in which to have your baby and to a hospital serving as backup for a birth-center or home birth.

   Whether the hospital will be safe depends in large part on the extent to which it provides four kinds of services:

- twenty-four-hour presence at the hospital of specialists in anesthesiology or of anesthetists,
- twenty-four-hour availability of blood from a bank at the hospital,
- twenty-four-hour availability of a complete operating-room staff, and
- twenty-four-hour availability of labor monitoring services including equipment and fully competent personnel for managing external and internal EFM, ultrasound scans, and fetal-scalp blood-sampling tests.

   Only in hospitals with a large maternity service or at major medical centers are you likely to find each of these services furnished to the extent listed above. Should such a hospital not be reasonably accessible to you, note to what extent—and especially with what timing, delays, and limitations—services of these kinds would be accessible at each of the available hospitals. Talk over your findings with your care-giver in deciding which hospital would be the most reasonable choice for you. If you are having a cesarean long planned in advance, for example, immediate availability of these services may not be very important since your surgery will be scheduled.

Your selection of a hospital should be made with care, too, if you are attempting a vaginal birth but may need an emergency cesarean because of previous cesareans or a chronic health problem.

Arranging for the Kind of Cesarean You Want

Many practitioners and hospitals in all parts of the country now offer significant alternatives in cesarean birth. These can go far toward making an unavoidable cesarean an essentially satisfying experience in which you have input on fundamental decisions.

Start as early as possible in your pregnancy to learn about cesareans and the options open to you. Do this even though the whole idea of cesarean, surgery, blood, and operating rooms may be repugnant to you. (These can be tolerated for important purposes, mothers learn.) In general, women who learn about cesareans in advance react in far more positive ways than women who go into their cesareans passive and ignorant, and often heartsick and terrified as well.

Start early to search out your alternatives for a possible cesarean with specific care-givers and hospitals in your locale. If you can, make these searches before selecting your prenatal care-giver.

Beyond acquainting yourself with all the essentials covered here, you and your partner will probably find it helpful to watch a film on cesarean birth as shown in many prenatal classes. Seeing such films can help clear away a sense of dread and can also help you to react in positive, cooperative ways through each step of a cesarean because you know what to expect. Constructive reactions can actually result in better physical well-being for yourself and your baby.

You and your partner can also develop better understanding of cesarean birth by getting in touch with one of the widespread self-help groups of parents who have had cesareans. Among them are numerous local chapters and affiliates of C-SEC, Inc., and the Cesarean Prevention Movement, Inc. (see Appendix A). Most send informational literature on request; some offer classes or meetings to help expectant parents avoid needless cesareans and prepare for needed ones. Meeting with members can be particularly useful if you definitely know you will need a cesarean or are likely to have one because of some factor in your physical condition.

Through the teachers of your regular prenatal classes you should also be able to get the names of a few parents who have had cesarean births. Talking with these parents about their experience should prove enlightening. Of course, your basic talks about a possible cesarean of your own would be with your care-giver and the teachers of your prenatal classes.

You really can make fundamentally important decisions about a possible cesarean birth—decisions affecting how you will feel about the birth and your child, as well as decisions affecting virtually every phase of the operation.

Anesthesia: You usually have five main choices of anesthesia in a cesarean birth. In order of their desirability for cesareans, they are:

1. epidural,
2. spinal,
3. local,
4. preoperative sedatives or analgesics given with any of the first three, and
5. general (often preceded by preoperative sedatives or analgesics).

The first two are sometimes called "epidural block" and "spinal block." They are also termed "conduction" or "regional" anesthesia, to differentiate them from "local," "inhalation," or "general" anesthesia. Spinal anesthesia tends to be used less often for cesarean birth today because of difficulty in controlling levels of anesthesia, hypotension (lowered blood pressure), and spinal headache.

Any one of numbers 1 through 3 listed above, administered correctly with no preoperative sedatives, leaves you wide awake and pain-free through and after the abdominal surgery of a cesarean. In fact, it leaves you pain-free long enough after the birth for you to bond with and start breastfeeding your baby if you are permitted to do so in the operating room.

Saying no to preoperative sedation will not compromise your or your baby's health. In fact, the less medication, the better for the baby's health. But if you're very fearful and tense at the thought of the cesarean, you might say yes. Or you might decide for general anesthesia, which makes you completely unconscious.

Before receiving either an epidural or a spinal anesthetic, you will usually be given intravenous fluids. This is done to increase the volume of blood and thus keep your blood pressure from dropping, a side effect of anesthesia.

The conduction anesthesias, epidural and spinal, are administered with you either sitting on the side of the operating table or lying on your left side with your lower back rounded. The anesthesia is given by an anesthesiologist or obstetrical physician into the area of your spinal cord and deadens feeling in your abdomen and legs. You are awake, but feel no discomfort and gradually regain feeling and use of your legs.

Local anesthesia is given into the abdominal wall and is rarely used today, although one practitioner's experience with its use is described in a book written by Christopher Norwood. (See Appendix B.) Just the abdominal area injected is deadened. Your legs are not affected and you are wide awake.

Sedatives or pain-relieving analgesics given to you before a cesarean represent minor calming medications rather than major anesthetics. However, it is very important for you to understand their effects.

General anesthesia is the fastest-acting and safest type for emergencies that involve very serious hemorrhaging of the mother or extreme fetal distress. It is available and familiar to the operating room staffs in almost every hospital.

Under general anesthesia, the woman is completely unconscious through the cesarean and for at least an hour after it—which some women see as an advantage and others view as a major disadvantage because it precludes active experience of the birth and bonding with and putting the baby to breast after the birth.

With general anesthesia there is a greater chance of depressive effects on the baby's system than with a spinal or epidural, if more than about ten minutes elapse between administration of anesthetic and delivery of the baby. (However, experienced obstetricians can often deliver a baby by cesarean section in less than five minutes after the first incision.)

Grogginess and sleepiness from the general anesthetic, though less likely today than in the past, may continue for a number of hours, and may be so extreme that you cannot wake up enough or focus to see (or to remember having seen) your baby when it is brought to you. Such grogginess clears up in half a day or so for some women, while for others it may decrease very slowly over several days.

Some women have nightmares or hallucinations, or cannot remember where they are or why, as they wake up after general anesthesia in the recovery room. Nurses will watch for and relieve such anxious or disoriented states, which usually end shortly.

The incision: It's legitimate for you to discuss the type of incision in the uterus you want for a first cesarean birth, unless there is an essential medical reason for having a certain one. The preferred type is the transverse low segment incision. Other types include the "classical incision"—a long vertical one that starts high on the uterus—and a shorter vertical one low on the uterus. These may be needed for some rare medical conditions. It is possible that a different incision is made in the skin and overlying tissues than in the uterus itself. Be sure to determine whether your physician care-giver uses that technique because a "classical" scar in the skin may not mean a "classical" incision into the uterus.

Your birth support partner: Decisions thus far have involved mainly your care-giver. This question and the following ones concern primarily your hospital.

First, at this hospital, is the father (or other support partner) permitted to be with you through the cesarean birth in the operating room? (Some permit only fathers.)

Second, could he or she stay with you or visit you in the room to which you would be taken after the operation to recover from the anesthesia?

You may have some difficulty finding a hospital that permits this practice and the following ones, which represent relatively new advances in family-centered care. You may have to search farther afield for a hospital meeting your requirements.

You're likely to be most interested in having these family-centered features of a cesarean birth if you plan on a type of anesthetic that leaves you conscious. However, some hospitals allow the father to be present even if the mother's condition requires general anesthesia. The couple's and the care-giver's view in cases like this is that the father can still reassure the mother, can give her a way of later learning about her own birth experience, and can carry out first bonding with the baby for them.

Hospitals in some cases have the father stand by outside the operating room while the mother is anesthetized, draped, and otherwise prepared for surgery. Fathers in all cases must "scrub" (wash their hands and forearms with antiseptic soap) and don operating-room gowns, caps, and surgical masks before entering the operating rooms, where they usually stand or sit by the mother's head. Drapes over a frame at her chest keep her from seeing any of the surgery. Fathers need not watch the surgery either, unless they wish to do so and are sure not to be upset by it.

Whether the father can be with the mother in the postoperative recovery room after the surgery represents a separate question for the hospital. You may find hospitals more reluctant to allow fathers in the recovery room than in the operating room because of the privacy of other patients there. In a large hospital, the recovery room can be crowded with many patients who need close watching and urgent care by the nurses, and patients are constantly being wheeled in and out. Moreover, patients are often only partially conscious because of anesthetics or pain-killers they've been given, and need to rest after their surgery.

Still, some hospitals permit fathers to be in the recovery room after cesareans, if only for a short time, and others permit fathers and/or babies in the recovery room but not in the operating room. Fathers are usually permitted entry if the hospital has a separate maternity recovery room (as is usually the case).

Bonding: You might also ask if the hospital's procedures permit some ten to thirty minutes for bonding with the baby right after birth. Bonding after cesareans is allowed in increasing numbers of hospitals.

Of course, you would be able to bond with the baby right after birth only if you had epidural or spinal anesthesia for the cesarean. With such regional anesthesia, you and your partner could carry out bonding while your incisions were being closed.

Hospital practices providing for bonding right after birth naturally require that the baby be in good health and condition, as most babies are who are born by cesarean after full forty-week pregnancies. Should your baby need constant observation or other urgent medical care right after birth, you can start bonding as soon as his or her health permits. Get your care-giver's support for bonding, in order to avoid misunderstanding or conflict.

If you will be allowed to bond, ask also to have any eye prophylaxis postponed until afterward. Delaying will in no way reduce the effectiveness of the medication, and will permit the unhindered eye contact important in bonding.

As part of bonding after a cesarean, you may also be able to nurse for a short time.

See if and where you may be permitted to bond with the baby after birth even if the father may not be allowed in the operating room; some hospitals permit mother-baby bonding in the recovery room but not the operating room.

"Gentle birth": You could also ask if at least some features of the Leboyer "gentle birth" can be provided after your cesarean birth. Increasing numbers of hospitals permit this as well, even though doing so in a hospital operating room will be more difficult than in a homelike birth room outfitted for normal vaginal birth.

Gentle birth features that might most readily be provided (in the absence of any urgent medical problems) include a warm "Leboyer bath" of the baby by the father (since you must continue to lie on your back), to go along with the reassurance of bonding, and a quiet atmosphere, with voices lowered and less clatter of instruments and equipment.

Rooming-in: For breastfeeding mothers especially, provision of rooming-in by hospitals has become increasingly common. Babies with no special health problems stay in a crib in the mother's room most of the time rather than in the infant nursery. This arrangement greatly facilitates breastfeeding, since the baby can be fed whenever it's hungry and need not be transported back and forth by a nurse.

Rooming-in can be adapted for mothers who have had a cesarean, as needed by their condition. Mothers usually must go through one or more days of postoperative recovery before they are strong enough and pain-free enough to move around and pick up the baby.

Breastfeeding: Even if the hospital does not provide for rooming-in, you might want to find out if its maternity-care practices encourage or discourage breastfeeding. Encouragement for cesarean mothers requires three practices:

• Bringing the baby to the mother from the nursery for breastfeeding every three or four hours, or more often if the baby's hungry, twenty-four hours a day;

• not routinely giving the baby bottles of formula or water in the nursery; and

• careful positioning of the mother and the baby to avoid incisional pain for the mother.

Special effort on the hospital's part may be needed for mothers who have had general anesthesia and who remain too sleepy or uncomfortable to nurse their babies for two or three days after the birth. In such cases, the hospital will start the baby on bottles but then switch to taking the baby to the mother as soon as she's able to nurse. Feeding at breast can be carried out even after a late start if you're persistent, confident, relaxed, and encouraged.

Father's visiting hours: Ask too if the father can visit you and the baby at any time over a span of many hours, such as 8 a.m to 10 p.m. daily. The father must be free of any illnesses like a cold and the mother and baby also should be in good health.

Sibling visits: Family-centered birth includes having a baby's brothers and sisters see their mother and the new sibling during or shortly after the birth. In choosing a hospital, ask about practices concerning such sibling visits with the mother after a cesarean.

Rising numbers of hospitals allow even very young children of cesarean mothers to visit—if not in the mother's own hospital room, then in a lounge on the maternity floor. Young children are also allowed to see the baby brother or sister through the glass of the nursery window. Some hospitals permit healthy new cesarean babies to be seen in the mother's room by young brothers and sisters who are in good health.

Alternatives like these will be available to you if you can find them at nearby hospitals and if your condition makes them medically feasible. Combine them as you can for the type of cesarean birth you would most prefer, in case you should need one.

You can arrange as many such alternatives as possible for a fully family-centered experience. Or you can set up a partly family-centered cesarean birth to include those alternatives that you decide are the most important ones.

Simplest of all to arrange would be a traditional cesarean birth with no family-centered features. However, as you realize, you don't have to settle for a traditional one unless you decide that's the kind you want. As with so many other vital elements in your childbearing experience, the main decisions today are yours.

Appendix A

~ ᴐ ᴄ ᴐ

Finding Maternity Services in Your Area

The International Childbirth Education Association is the best single source of services available to you in your locality. We have added some additional organizations which may be of specific assistance. The ICEA was founded in 1960, in part as an outgrowth of work by the Maternity Center Association in the 1940s and 1950s in fostering informed childbearing and especially "natural childbirth."

A. PRENATAL CLASSES

Referrals to classes given by childbirth educators may be requested from:

American Academy of Husband-Coached Childbirth (Bradley/Dick-Read)
P.O. Box 5224
Sherman Oaks, CA 91413

American Society for Psychoprophylaxis in Obstetrics (Lamaze)
1840 Wilson Blvd., Suite 204
Arlington, VA 22201

Childbirth Without Pain Education Association (Lamaze)
20134 Snowden
Detroit, MI 48235

International Childbirth Education Association (All types)
P.O. Box 20048
Minneapolis, MN 55420

Maternity Center Association (All types)
48 E. 92nd Street
New York, NY 10128

Read Natural Childbirth Foundation (Dick-Read)
1300 S. Eliseo Dr., Suite 102
Greenbrae, CA 94904

B. BREASTFEEDING SUPPORT GROUPS

La Leche League International
9616 Minneapolis Ave.
Franklin Park, IL 60131

C. BIRTH BY CESAREAN SECTION GROUPS

Cesarean Prevention Movement
P.O. Box 152
Syracuse, NY 13210
(chapters in major regions of the country)

C/SEC (Cesareans/Support, Education, and Concern)
22 Forest Rd.
Framingham, MA 01701

The Cesarean Connection
P.O. Box 11
Westmont, IL 60559

D. ALTERNATIVE BIRTH SETTINGS IN GENERAL

American College of Nurse-Midwives
1522 K Street N.W.
Suite 1120
Washington, D.C. 20005

International Association of Parents and Professionals for Safe Alternatives
in Childbirth
P.O. Box 267
Marble Hill, MO 63764

National Association of Childbearing Centers
Box 1, Route 1
Perkiomenville, PA 18074

E. GENETICS ORGANIZATIONS

General guidance on the likelihood of your unborn baby having a
hereditary or other type of birth defect can be provided by many profes-

sionals experienced in prenatal care. Information of this kind may also be obtained by writing to the National Genetics Foundation (555 W. 57th St., New York, NY 10019). Staff members there will send you general information and a "Family Health Profile" form; if you fill this out, the Foundation will analyze it for a small charge. (The Foundation serves as a national referral source to genetic counseling centers.)

You might also inquire at your local chapter of the March of Dimes for lists of qualified centers. This organization does not offer any screening or advisory services to the public. Rather, it supports research and public information programs that seek to reduce birth defects.

Appendix B

ᕗᐁᑕᕋᐁᑕᐁᐧᕋ

Additional Sources of Information

Readers who want further information may find it helpful to consult some of the publications listed here. These are selected listings reprinted with permission from *Bookmarks* for May 1985 (with the exception of added works published by the Maternity Center Association).

Bookmarks is the thrice-yearly published bulletin of the ICEA Bookcenter, which is operated by the International Childbirth Education Association to serve as a comprehensive and reliable source of books and pamphlets on childbirth preparation, family-centered maternity care, and related family and professional subjects.

A complete current listing of these and other publications that can be ordered from the ICEA will be sent in response to a request accompanied by a stamped (37¢), self-addressed, no. 10 envelope mailed to ICEA Bookcenter, P.O. Box 20048, Minneapolis, MN 55420-0048. This is also the mailing address for *Bookmarks,* for which Doris T. Olson is the editor.

Books are listed in alphabetic order by titles.

PREGNANCY, BIRTH, AND CHILDBIRTH PREPARATION

Assertive Childbirth: The Future Parent's Guide to a Positive Pregnancy, Susan Mckay, trade paperback, 1983. Provides accurate, timely information on childbirth alternatives and explains exactly how to get the type you want.

Birth Atlas, 6th ed., Maternity Center Association, easel-back book. Includes photographic reproductions of the classic Dickenson-Belski sculptures that depict fertilization, development of the embryo and fetus, and labor and birth. The process is thoroughly explained in the accompanying text. A classic work, used and recommended by childbirth educators throughout the world.

Birth Over Thirty, Sheila Kitzinger, trade paperback, 1985. Designed to help the pregnant woman over 30 understand what is happening to her, how to take an active part in her pregnancy and birth, and how to cope with the challenges before and after the birth.

Birthrights, Sally Inch, trade paperback, 1984. Provides critical, step-by-step review of interventions used routinely in hospital childbirth: why things are done and the risks and benefits.

Birth—Through Children's Eyes, Sandra VanDam Anderson, and Penny Simkin, trade paperback, 1981. An examination of children's perceptions of the childbirth process, including cesarean births; prenatal preparation suggestions for children. Well illustrated.

Birth Without Violence, Frederick Leboyer, hardcover, 1975. Making birth more peaceful for the vulnerable, sensitive newborn. Poetic and powerful, with remarkable photographs. A classic by the originator of "gentle birth."

Bonding: How Parents Become Attached to Their Baby, Diony Young, pamphlet, 1978. Focuses on the importance of early establishment of the parent-infant bond and factors that affect this attachment process.

Bonding: The Beginnings of Parent-Infant Attachment, rev. ed., Marshall Klaus and John Kennell, trade paperback, 1983. Revision of a classic work on bonding; issued in former editions under the title *Parent-Infant Bonding.*

Changing Childbirth: Family Birth in the Hospital, Diony Young, trade paperback, 1982. Substantial, thoughtful book discusses needs of the family, including siblings, in childbirth; benefits of family-centered care; birth companions; birthing rooms and birthing centers; family-centered cesarean birth; and childbirth education.

Childbirth With Insight, Elizabeth Noble, trade paperback, 1983. Encourages expectant parents to use the months of pregnancy to develop the self-reliance and personal responsibility to plan their own birth experience.

Childbirth Without Fear, 4th ed., Grantley Dick-Read, mass paperback, 1972. This edition, revised by Wessel & Ellis, incorporates the best of the late Dick-Read's writings, principles, and practice, and his biography. A classic by the obstetrician who in large part originated natural childbirth several decades ago.

A Child Is Born, Lennert Nilsson, hardcover, 1977. Human reproduction from conception to birth as portrayed extensively in outstanding color photographs, taken in many cases inside the body by remarkable microphotographic techniques.

The Complete Book of Pregnancy and Childbirth, Sheila Kitzinger, hardcover, 1980. Comprehensive guide to pregnancy and childbirth fully illustrated with photographs, drawings, and diagrams.

Entering the World: The De-Medicalization of Childbirth, Michel Odent, hardcover and paperback, 1984. English translation of Odent's book *Bien Naître.* Focuses on allowing the birth of a baby to be a welcoming continuation of the feelings and rhythms of the womb.

Essential Exercises for the Childbearing Year, 2nd ed., Elizabeth Noble, trade paperback, 1982. Guide to understanding the changes of pregnancy with ways to assist the woman in dealing with them.

Ever Since Eve: Personal Reflections on Childbirth, Nancy Caldwell Sorel, hardcover, 1984. Reactions about birth experiences from women around the world—rich and poor, contemporary and historic; shows the childbirth experience as always unique yet essentially the same for all.

Giving Birth, Mary M. Kalergis, trade paperback, 1983. Beautiful, moving photo journal, captioned by direct quotes of those in each photograph; striking black and white photos show numerous facets of childbirth in a memorable way.

A Good Birth, A Safe Birth, Diana Korte and Roberta Scaer, trade paperback, 1984. Includes survey results of women's childbearing preferences and explanation of available childbirth options.

Guide to Family-Centered Childbirth, Donna and Roger Ewy, trade paperback, 1981. Details new developments in Lamaze method, family-centered alternatives, anatomy and physiology, processes of labor and delivery, relaxation and breathing, comfort measures, possible problems and interventions, and cesarean birth.

Having a Baby After Thirty, Elisabeth Bing and Libby Colman, mass paperback, 1980. Answers to most frequently asked questions concerning how age affects childbirth.

Having Twins, A Parent's Guide to Pregnancy, Birth, and Early Parenthood, Elizabeth Noble, trade paperback, 1980. Prenatal care, parenting tips, and fascinating facts dealing with multiple births.

Husband-Coached Childbirth, 3rd ed., Robert Bradley, hardcover, 1981. Detailed description of the Bradley method of husband-coached childbirth, by the method's originator.

Immaculate Deception: A New Look at Women and Childbirth, Suzanne Arms, mass paperback, 1977. Exploration of the warping of childbirth in modern times.

In a Family Way, Susan Lapinski and Michael DeCourcy Hinds, hardcover, 1982. A husband and wife's diary of everything from the decision to have a child through pregnancy, birth, and their first year as new parents.

Managing Your Maternity Leave, Meg Wheatley and Marcie Schorr Hirsch, trade paperback, 1983. Explains planning and negotiating maternity leave, staying visible while on leave, and reentering the organization.

The Maternity Sourcebook, Wendy and Matthew Lesko, trade paperback, 1984. Exhaustive exploration of factors in childbirth and early child care to help parents make their own decisions concerning pregnancy, delivery, and baby care.

Methods of Childbirth, 2nd ed., Constance A. Bean, trade paperback, 1982. Comprehensive new edition of a guide for expectant parents with current discussion summarizing alternative approaches to prenatal care and childbirth.

Newborn Needs: Maternity Center Association, 1986–Booklet designed for parents who elect short stay programs.

The New Our Bodies, Ourselves, Boston Women's Health Book Collective, trade paperback, 1984. A comprehensive reading on the biological and psychological functioning of women.

The Pregnancy After 30 Workbook, Gail Sforza Brewer, Ed., trade paperback, 1978. Encourages expectant mothers to use exercise, self-awareness, and diet to help ensure a healthy pregnancy, a problem-free birth, and an easy postpartum period.

Pregnancy & Childbirth: The Complete Guide for a New Life, Tracy Hotchner, trade paperback, 1984. Examines alternatives and their physical and emotional consequences.

Pregnancy and Life-Style Habits, Peter A. Fried, trade paperback, 1983. Presents the facts about the effects of alcohol, caffeine, nicotine, marijuana, and prescription and over-the-counter drugs on the unborn baby.

Pregnancy, Childbirth, and the Newborn, Penny Simkin, Janet Whalley, and Ann Keppler, trade paperback, 1984. Covers nutrition, prenatal procedures, health-care providers, birth places, labor support techniques, medical interventions, exercises, relaxation, and breast-feeding, with strong presentation of parental choice and excellent charts.

The Pregnant Patient's Bill of Rights—The Pregnant Patient's Responsibilities, Doris Haire and members of ICEA, no date, pamphlet. Contains the statement by the American College of Obstetricians and Gynecologists in support of informed consent by the patient, as well as a listing of the patient's responsibilities.

Premature Babies—A Handbook for Parents, rev. ed., Sherri Nance, mass paperback, 1984. A step-by-step explanation of the emotional obstacles encountered by parents of premature babies, with sharing of experiences of other parents.

The Premature Baby Book, Helen Harrison and Ann Kositzky, trade paperback, 1983. Deals with emotions, bonding, and parenting in the nursery, causes of the early delivery and techniques to prevent it, feeding and nutrition; lists over 100 support groups and national organizations.

Preparation for Childbearing, rev. 5th ed., Maternity Center Association, booklet, 1985. A popular, thoroughly illustrated booklet that offers practical suggestions with specific exercises to increase comfort during pregnancy and to prepare for labor. Also included are full explanations of breathing and relaxation techniques to use during labor and birth. Advice also on the postpartum period and breastfeeding, and hints for the expectant father.

The Secret Life of the Unborn Child, Thomas Verny and John Kelly, trade paperback, 1981. Based on two decades of medical research; presents ways the unborn baby responds to prenatal influences.

Six Practical Lessons for an Easier Childbirth, rev. ed., Elisabeth Bing, trade paperback, 1982. Step-by-step guide to the Lamaze method of childbirth, extensively illustrated.

Thank You, Dr. Lamaze, rev. ed., Marjorie Karmel, trade paperback, 1983. Classic work largely responsible for the widespread introduction of the Lamaze method in the United States, written for other expectant couples by a young American who went to France with her husband to have their baby delivered by Dr. Lamaze himself.

Transformation Through Birth, A Women's Guide, Claudia Panuthos, trade paperback, 1984. Heralds childbirth movement's passing into stronger, holistic period; chapters on preparation for birth using visualization and release.

Twins, From Conception to Five Years, Averil Clegg and Anne Woollett, trade paperback, 1983. Guides the reader through genetics, pregnancy, preparation, labor, postpartum, nourishment and child care; stresses the importance of emotional support and suggests where to get it.

The Whole Birth Catalog, Janet Isaacs Ashford, Ed., trade paperback, 1983. Comprehensive consumer's guide in the style and format of *The Whole Earth Catalog,* treating pregnancy and birth and including reviews of books and pamphlets and descriptions of products, resources, and organizations; extensive illustrations.

CESAREAN BIRTH

Cesarean Childbirth: A Handbook for Parents, Christine Coleman Wilson and Wendy Roe Hoven, trade paperback, 1981. Invaluable resource for couples seeking to prepare themselves for all possibilities of childbirth; contents range from trends and issues in obstetrics to parent-infant bonding.

Guide for Cesarean Births, C/SEC, trade paperback, 1983. Guide to what can be expected during a cesarean birth and available options.

How to Avoid a Cesarean Section, Christopher Norwood, hardcover, 1984. Explains strategies used to avert unneeded surgery and steps available to get best medical care if surgery is needed.

Silent Knife: Cesarean Prevention and Vaginal Birth After Cesarean, Nancy Wainer Cohen and Lois J. Estner, trade paperback, 1983. Very comprehensive information to increase consumer awareness of this complex medical procedure, written with humor as well as some indignation.

BREASTFEEDING

Breastfeeding, Janice Presser, Gail Sforza Brewer, and Julianna FreeHand, hardcover, 1983. Provides guidance on everything from how to begin nursing to ways of weaning; fully illustrated.

Breastfeeding Basics, Cecilia Worth, trade paperback, 1983. Easy-to-read guide for the busy breastfeeding mother, explaining the how and why of breastfeeding; relaxed, friendly, and direct tone; fully illustrated.

The Breastfeeding Book, Maire Messenger, trade paperback, 1982. Provides facts, practical information, and guidance to help make breastfeeding as simple, enjoyable, and successful as possible; well illustrated.

Breastfeeding: How to Succeed, Derek Llewellyn-Jones, trade paperback, 1983. How lactation occurs, how it is established and maintained, and answers to questions asked by breastfeeding mothers.

Breastfeeding Twins, Triplets, and Quadruplets: 195 Practical Hints for Success, Donald M. Keith et al., Eds., trade paperback, 1982. Practical methods and suggestions for women who wish to simultaneously breastfeed two or more infants, based on experiences of mothers who have breastfed their multiples; collected by the Parents Multiple Birth Associations of Canada.

The Womanly Art of Breastfeeding, 3rd ed., La Leche League International, trade paperback, 1981. A classic; practical manual by the organization that for two decades has been offering instruction and support to nursing mothers.

PARENTHOOD

Congratulations! You're Going to Be a Grandmother, Lanie Carter, hardcover/paperback, 1980. Emphasizes the grandmother's role in enhancing a new family's bonding, spells out pitfalls, and gives specific ways for a grandmother to be most helpful.

The Grandparents' Handbook, Hugh Jolly, trade paperback, 1984. Provides a refresher course for grandparents with information on coping with emergencies, child-proofing the house and yard, and having an all-around good time with grandchildren.

Guide to Parenting: You and Your Newborn, Donna and Roger Ewy, trade paperback, 1981. Provides information on the importance of family bonding; newborn characteristics; common concerns of parenthood; postnatal exercises and health care; changing parental roles; marriage and sexuality.

Of Cradles and Careers: A Guide to Reshaping Your Job to Include a Baby in Your Life, Kay Lowman, trade paperback, 1984.

An excellent how-to book on structuring time and job responsibilities to allow for baby's need for mother's time.

Pregnant Fathers, Jack Heinowitz, trade paperback, 1982. Examines the feelings, needs, and concerns of expectant and new fathers.

Welcoming Your Second Baby, Vicki Lansky, mass paperback, 1984. Provides effective ways to help the second baby fit into the family.

What Now? A Handbook for New Parents, Mary Lou Rozdilsky and Barbara Banet, trade paperback, 1975. Covers all facets of the adjustments to parenthood.

Your Second Child, Joan Solomon Weiss, trade paperback, 1981. Gives a detailed look at the impact of a second child on the family, discusses psychological and physical aspects of a second pregnancy and childbirth, and offers information on coping with sibling rivalry, differences between children, and other concerns.

INFANT CARE

Circumcision: The Painful Dilemma, Rosemary Romberg, trade paperback, 1985. Thoroughly researched and balanced critique of current medical research, myths, and realities; extensive bibliography and glossary.

Crying Baby, Sleepless Nights, Sandy Jones, trade paperback, 1983. Comprehensive guide to many causes of infant crying, including practical, unique suggestions for coping with emotions and making the baby more comfortable.

Dr. Spock's Baby and Child Care, Benjamin Spock and Michael B. Rothenberg, hardcover, 1985. Revised edition of a classic.

The First Three Years of Life, Burton L. White, trade paperback, 1978. A detailed guide to the development of the young child.

First-Year Baby Care, Paula Kelly, Ed., trade paperback, 1983. Illustrated step-by-step guide for new parents, covering bathing, diapering, feeding, medical emergencies, and developmental milestones.

On Becoming A Family, T. Berry Brazelton, trade paperback, 1982. This book traces the process of attachment, starting with the feelings of the pregnant mother and father-to-be through the first days at home and later weeks when the attachment becomes reciprocal and the baby and parents settle into each other's rhythms.

The Parents' Guide to Baby and Child Medical Care, Terril H. Hart, Ed., looseleaf, 1983. Easy to use step-by-step instructions for the treatment of over 105 common children's illnesses, injuries, and emergencies; includes an index of symptoms, illness and immunization record forms, anatomy charts, height/weight charts, medicine chest checklist, and accident prevention and child-proofing tips.

The Premature Baby Book: A Parent's Guide to Coping and Caring in the First Years, Helen Harrison and Ann Kositsky, trade paperback, 1983. Believing that only parents of sick infants can really understand and communicate with others in the same situation, the authors have used interviews with parents and medical personnel to explain the effects of prematurity on the child, family, and care-givers.

The Well Baby Book, Mike Samuels and Nancy Samuels, trade paperback, 1979. Underscores preventive medicine in a guide to child care from conception to age 4.

DEALING WITH GRIEF

After a Loss in Pregnancy, Nancy Berezin, trade paperback, 1982. Based on hundreds of interviews with women who have experienced miscarriages, stillbirths, or neonatal deaths, this book not only describes their thoughts and emotions but explains stages and symptoms of grief; includes listing of parent support groups and a bibliography.

Ended Beginnings—Healing Childbearing Losses, Claudia Panuthos and Catherine Romeo, trade paperback, 1984. A healing book showing parents how to use inner resources to grieve successfully for the loss of a child—through miscarriage, stillbirth, sudden infant death, or abortion; also treats subsequent adoption.

When Pregnancy Fails, Susan Borg and Judith Lasker, trade paperback, 1981. Written for families coping with miscarriage, stillbirth, and infant death, and for the professionals who help them.

FOOD AND NUTRITION

As You Eat, So Your Baby Grows, Nikki Goldbeck, booklet, 1980. A guide to nutrition during pregnancy.

The Brewer Medical Diet for Normal and High-Risk Pregnancy, Gail Sforza Brewer and Thomas Brewer, trade paperback, 1983. Provides specific, proper nutritional program for every stage during and after pregnancy, from conception to weaning.

Nourishing Your Unborn Child, Phyllis Williams, trade paperback, 1982. A guide to nutrition during pregnancy and postpartum, with menus and recipes.

Nutrition for the Childbearing Year, Jacqueline Gibson Gazella, ringbound, 1979. Basic information on essential nutrients during pregnancy and breastfeeding, including menus and recipes.

Nutrition for Your Pregnancy, Judith E. Brown, trade paperback, 1983. University of Minnesota guide containing scientific information about nutrition and pregnancy, written in upbeat supportive tone.

Nutrition in Pregnancy and Lactation, 3rd ed., Worthington-Roberts and Vermeersch & Williams, trade paperback, 1985. Includes all aspects of maternal nutrition.

Pickles and Ice Cream, Mary Abbott Hess and Ann Elise Hunt, hardcover, 1982. A comprehensive guide to prenatal nutrition written in a warm and enjoyable style; covers common problems of nutrition in pregnancy and dispels myths.

Pregnancy and Nutrition: The Complete Guide and Calendar for D.I.E.T. During Pregnancy 1985–1986, Miriam Erick, looseleaf, 1984. This mini nutrition book helps to Develop Intelligent Eating Techniques (D.I.E.T.).

FOR CHILDREN

Daniel's Question, A Cesarean Birth Story, Elaine Sussman Allinson, booklet, 1981. Provides a simple clarification of the whys and wherefores of cesarean birth; suitable for 6- to 8-year-olds. Nicely illustrated.

I Want To Tell You About My Baby, Roslyn Banish, trade paperback, 1982. A book for children on coping with feelings when a new baby joins the family; charmingly illustrated.

Mom, Dad and I are Having a Baby, rev. ed., Maryann Malecki, trade paperback, 1982. A picture book that prepares children of all ages to be present at a birth.

Nobody Asked Me If I Wanted A Baby Sister, Martha Alexander, trade paperback, 1971. Oliver decides to give away his new baby sister because he's jealous, but in the end finds he really likes her after all; cute illustrations.

When The New Baby Comes I'm Moving Out, Martha Alexander, trade paperback, 1979. A humorous cartoon-style book on a little boy's feelings about his mother's pregnancy.

Notes

INTRODUCTION

1. Diony Young, *Changing Childbirth: Family Birth in the Hospital* (Rochester, NY: Childbirth Graphics Ltd., 1982), page ix. The full passage from which the quotation is taken reads:

"*Changing Childbirth*, the book, has been evolving during the same decade that has witnessed an extraordinary humanistic and technological revolution in obstetrical and newborn care. During the 1970s the literature and documentation in support of family-centered maternity care has become increasingly voluminous. Finally the time came to gather it all together and put it in one book so it would be readily available to health providers, childbirth educators, and consumers when they needed it. . . ."

CHAPTER 4

1. Sharron Hannon, *Childbirth* (New York: M. Evans & Co., 1980), p. 90.

2. American Academy of Pediatrics/The American College of Obstetricians and Gynecologists *Guidelines for Perinatal Care* (Washington, D.C.: American College of Obstetricians and Gynecologists, 1983), p. 166. (Joint publisher: Evanston, IL: American Academy of Pediatrics, 1983.)

3. Food and Nutrition Board, National Academy of Sciences–National Research Council, *Recommended Dietary Allowances, Ninth Edition,* Washington, DC: National Academy Press, 1980.

4. Committee on Dietary Allowances, Food and Nutrition Board *Recommended Dietary Allowances,* 9th ed. (Washington, DC: National Academy of Sciences, 1980), p. 5.

317

CHAPTER 5

1. Developed by Dr. Ilya Spigland, chief of the division of virology at Montefiori Medical Center in New York, use of this procedure had begun to spread to other diagnostic facilities in 1986. Dr. Spigland is also associate professor of pediatrics at Albert Einstein College of Medicine.

CHAPTER 9

1. Sylvia Feldman, *Choices in Childbirth* (New York: Grosset and Dunlap, 1978), p. 7.

2. A. D. Haverkamp, H. E. Thompson, J. G. McFee, *et al.*, "The Evaluation of Continuous Fetal Heart Rate Monitoring in High-Risk Pregnancy," *American Journal of Obstetrics and Gynecology* 125(1976):310–20.

A. D. Haverkamp, M. Orleans, and J. R. Murphy, "The Differential Effects of Fetal Monitoring on Mothers and Infants." Presented at the meetings of the American Public Health Association, Washington, DC, October 1977 (unpublished).

3. J. A. Lowe, D. F. Klassen, and R. J. Loup, "Cesarean Sections in U.S. PAS [Professional Activity Study] Hospitals," *PAS Reporter* 14(1976):1.

4. A. D. Haverkamp, "Home Delivery vs. Fetal Monitoring," *Report of 1977 National Health Forum: The Third Century—Resource Limits and the Trade-Offs in Developing America's Health Policy.* New York: The Forum, March 1977, p. 49.

5. M. L. Romney, "Predelivery Shaving: An Unjustified Assault?" *Journal of Obstetrics and Gynecology,* 1(1980):33–35.

6. M. L. Romney and G. Gordon, "Is Your Enema Really Necessary?" *British Medical Journal* 282(1981):1269–71.

7. National Institutes of Health, *Cesarean Childbirth (Consensus Development Conference Summary, Vol. 3, No. 6)* (Bethesda, MD: U.S. Department of Health and Human Services, 1981).

8. Diony Young, "Policy Reversal for Vaginal Delivery After Cesarean," *ICEA News,* May 1982.

9. American College of Obstetricians and Gynecologists, "Vaginal Delivery After Cesarean" (Washington, D.C.). News release, Feb. 24, 1982.

10. J. A. Lowe, D. F. Klassen, and R. J. Loop, *op. cit.*

11. American College of Obstetricians and Gynecologists, Committee on Obstetrics, *Maternal and Fetal Medicine: Guidelines for Vaginal Delivery After a Cesarean Childbirth* (Washington, DC, 1982).

12. B. Jordan, *Birth in Four Cultures: A Crosscultural Investigation of Childbirth in Yucatan, Holland, Sweden and the United States* (St. Albans, VT: Eden Press Women's Publications, 1978).

13. R. W. Lubic, *Barriers and Conflict in Maternity Care Innovation.* Dissertation submitted in partial fulfillment of the requirements for the Ed.D.

degree at Teachers College, Columbia University, New York, NY, 1979 (unpublished).

14. Ibid.

15. Committee on Assessing Alternative Birth Settings, Institute of Medicine, National Academy of Sciences, *Research Issues in the Assessment of Birth Settings* (Washington, DC: National Academy Press, 1982).

CHAPTER 11

1. Popularly reported on in "Study Cites Sharp Increase in Breast Feeding," *The New York Times,* March 25, 1984, p. 31.

CHAPTER 13

1. "New Restrictions on Oxytocin Use," *FDA Drug Bulletin* (1978). See also E. E. Nichols, "Guidelines for Induction of Labor," *JAMA* 245 (1981), p. 777–78.

CHAPTER 14

1. Marshall H. Klaus and John H. Kennell, *Parent-Infant Bonding,* 2nd ed. (St. Louis: Mosby, 1982).

2. Frederick Leboyer, *Birth Without Violence* (New York: Knopf, 1975).

CHAPTER 17

0. A. Haverkamp, et al., "Differential Effects of Intrapartum Fetal Monitoring," *American Journal of Obstetrics and Gynecology* 134 (1979): 399–408.

1. Norbert Gleicher, "Cesarean Section Rates in the United States: The Short-Term Failure of the National Consensus Development Conference in 1980," *JAMA* 252 (1984): 3273–76.

2. Richard Hausknecht and Joan Rattner Heilman, *Having a Cesarean Baby,* 2nd ed. (New York: Dutton, 1982), p. 193.

3. See Chapter 9, note 7.

4. Ibid.

5. H. Haesslein and K. Niswander, "Fetal Distress in Term Pregnancies," *American Journal of Obstetrics and Gynecology* 137 (1980): 245.

Index

Hazards, 55–64
(*See also* Precautions)
Head, baby, 240–241
Head and shoulders lift exercise, 144–145
Heart disease, cesarean section and, 289
Heartburn, 66
Hemorrhoids, 66–67, 72
Herbicides, 61
Herpes simplex virus II, 62–63
Hexachlorophene, 59
Hiccups, 249
High blood pressure, cesarean section and, 289
Home birth, 108–112
 finding care-givers for, 128
 precautions for, 111–112
 preparation for, 193
Home preparation, 188–191
 clothes in, 190–191
 equipment in, 188–190
 furniture in, 188–190
 home birth and, 193
 supplies in, 190–191
Home-use pregnancy tests, 15–16
Hospitals:
 birth in, 246
  conventional, 117–119
  humanized, 115–117
 breastfeeding in, 173
 cesarean section and, 292–295
 choosing of: cesarean section and, 292–295
  family-centered maternity care and, 127
  traditional hospital birth and, 128
 family-centered maternity care in, 127
 finding care-givers for, 129
 labor and delivery in, 230–234
 traditional hospital birth in, 128
Hot chocolate, 56
Hot tubs, 64
Hydramnios, 276
Hygiene, personal, 255

Illness of babies, 262–263
Immature labor, 273
Inborn reflexes, 238
Incisions, cesarean section and, 298
Incompatibility, Rh, 281–282
Induced labor, 206–209
Infections, 61–63
Injury, avoidance of, 55–64
Intercourse:
 postnatal, 258–259
 prenatal, 32–33, 63–64
Inverted nipples, 172
Iron supplements, 42–43

Jaundice, 261–262
Junk food, 42

Kegel exercise, 143–144

Labor and delivery, 197–234
 abnormal, 278–279
 advance signs of, 209–210
 conventional hospital management of, 230–234

Labor and delivery (*cont.*)
 delay in, 279
 delivery in, 226–227, 230
 early, 211–213
 emergency childbirth in, 211–212
 false labor in, 209
 first-stage, 213–221
  breathing for, 153–156
 forceps-assisted deliveries in, 284–286
 immature, 273
 induced, 206–208
 late, 205–209
 preparations for, 202–204
 preterm, 267–269, 273
 prodromal, 278
 second-stage, 223–226, 228–230
  breathing for, 157–160
 start of, 210–211
 teamwork in, 212–213
 third-stage, 228–232
  breathing for, 160
 transition, 220–223
  breathing for, 156–157
Lanugo, 240
Late births, 205–209
Latent phase, prolonged, 278
LBW (low-birth-weight) babies, 39–40
Leboyer birth, 117
(*See also* Bonding; Gentle birth)
Leg cramps, 68
Leg spread exercise, 142–143
Lifting, 91–93
Lightening, 102, 197–199
Lightheadedness, 95
Liquid meals, 49–50
Lochia, 255–256
Looped cord, 280
Low-birth-weight (LBW) babies, 39–40
Lying down, 93–96

Massage, 152
 breast, 170–171
Maternity services, finding of, 303–305
Medications, 57
 breastfeeding and, 165
Menstrual period, missed, 14
Mercury, 59
Middle pregnancy, 85–97
(*See also* Second trimester)
Midwives (*see* Care-givers)
Milk, 43
 expressing, 171
 increasing supply of, 177–178
Mineral supplements for babies, 180
Miscarriage, 273–275
Mongolism (*see* Down syndrome)
Mood swings:
 in first trimester, 30–34
 postnatal, 258
 in third trimester, 102–105
Morning sickness:
 breakfast muffins for, 50–51
 remedy for, 65–66
 as sign of pregnancy, 14
Mucus, 72–73
Multiple fetuses, early detection of, 76–77
Muscle aches, abdominal, 69–70

Risks:
of advanced technology, 10
and hazards (*see* Precautions)
Rooming-in, 117
cesarean section and, 300
Rooting, 238
Rubella, 61
Rupture of membranes, 210
first-stage labor and, 154

Safety precautions (*see* Precautions)
Saliva, excess, 67
Salt, 42
swelling and, 74
Saunas, 64
Second-stage labor, 223–226, 228–230
breathing for, 157–160
guide for, 223–224
pushing positions in, 159
signs of, 157–158
transition to, 220–223
Second trimester, 85–97
body handling in, 89–95
emotions in, 95–97
fifth month of, 86–87
fourteenth week of, 85–86
lifting in, 91–93
posture in, 89–91
sixth month of, 88–89
sleeping positions in, 92–96
standing in, 89–91
third month of, 85–86
Section (*see* Cesarean sections)
Selective relaxation, 150
Sexual intercourse:
postnatal, 258–259
prenatal, 32–33, 63–64
Sexually transmitted diseases, 62–63
Shaving of pubic hair, 120–121
Short cord, 280
Shortness of breath, 67–68, 87
Shoulder circle exercise, 146–147
Show, 210
Siblings (*see* Children)
Silver nitrate, 242
Skin:
baby, 240
maternal, changes in, 73–74
Sleepiness, 67–68
Sleeping:
babies and, 249–250
during pregnancy, positions for, 92–96
Smoking, 56
Snacks, 49
Solid foods, 176–177
Solvents, 60
Spitting up, 249
Spontaneous abortion, 273–275
Sports, 64
Squat exercise, 145–146
Stages of labor (*see* Labor and delivery)
Stair climbing, 89–91
Standing, 89–91
Startle reflex, 238
Station, 214
Stepping reflex, 238
Stools of babies, 248–249
Stooping, 91–93

Stretch marks, 73
Supplements for babies:
mineral, 180
vitamin, 177, 180
Supplies, baby, 190–191
Support groups, choosing, 21
Support partner, cesarean section and, 298–299
Swelling, 74
in third trimester, 101
toxemia and, 270
Syntocinon, 208
Syphilis, 62

Tailor-sitting exercises, 141–143
Tay-Sachs disease, testing for, 77–80
Tea, 56
Teamwork, 160, 254
labor and delivery and, 212–213
Technology:
appropriate use of, 75–83
risks in use of, 10
(*See also* Tests)
Tests, 75–83
amniocentesis, 77–80
chorionic villus biopsy, 79–80
contraction stress, 82–83
electronic fetal monitoring, 80–83
nonstress, 80–81
oxytocin challenge, 82–83
pregnancy, 13–17
home-use, 15–16
laboratory, 15–17
ultrasound scan, 76–77
Third-stage labor, 228–232
breathing for, 160
Third trimester, 99–105
eighth month of, 99–102
emotional changes in, 102–105
ninth month of, 102–103
Tiredness, 67–68
in third trimester, 104
Tobacco, 56
Toluene, 60
Touch relaxation, 151–152
Toxemia, 269–271
Toxoplasmosis, 61–62
Tranquilizers, 56
breastfeeding and, 165
Transition, 220–223
breathing for, 156–157
signs of, 156–157
Transverse presentation, 277–278
Tubal pregnancy, 275–276
Turpentine, 60
Twins, early detection of, 76–77

Ultrasound scans, 76–77
date of birth and, 18
risk and, 10
Umbilical cord:
care of, 261
complications with, 280–281
cutting of, 239
Uranium wastes, 60
Urinary infections, 67
Urinary problems, Kegel exercise for, 143–144